# ■ GETTING
# ■ OLD
# WITHOUT
# GETTING
# ANXIOUS

■ ■ ■

## PETER V. RABINS, M.D.,

### WITH LYNN LAUBER

AVERY ■ A MEMBER OF PENGUIN GROUP (USA) INC. ■ NEW YORK

Published by the Penguin Group
www.penguin.com
Penguin Group (USA) Inc., 375 Hudson Street, New York, New York 10014, USA • Penguin Group (Canada),
90 Eglinton Avenue East, Suite 700, Toronto, Ontario M4P 2Y3, Canada (a division of Pearson Penguin Canada
Inc.) • Penguin Books Ltd, 80 Strand, London WC2R 0RL, England • Penguin Ireland, 25 St Stephen's Green,
Dublin 2, Ireland (a division of Penguin Books Ltd) • Penguin Group (Australia), 250 Camberwell Road, Camberwell,
Victoria 3124, Australia (a division of Pearson Australia Group Pty Ltd) • Penguin Books India Pvt Ltd, 11
Community Centre, Panchsheel Park, New Delhi–110 017, India • Penguin Group (NZ), Cnr Airborne and
Rosedale Roads, Albany, Auckland 1310, New Zealand (a division of New Zealand Ltd) • Penguin Books (South
Africa) (Pty) Ltd, 24 Sturdee Avenue, Rosebank, Johannesburg 2196, South Africa

Penguin Books Ltd, Registered Offices: 80 Strand, London WC2R 0RL, England

First trade papberback edition 2006

The Library of Congress cataloged the hardcover as follows:

Rabins, Peter V.   000174
  Getting old without getting anxious : conquering late-life anxiety / Peter V. Rabins with
Lynn Lauber.
    p.   cm.
  Includes bibliographical references.
  ISBN 1-58333-210-3
  1. Geriatric psychiatry.   2. Depression in old age.   3. Anxiety.
4. Older persons—Mental health.   I. Lauber, Lynn.   II. Title.
RC451.4.A5R336     2005               2004055126
618.97'689—dc22
ISBN: 1-58333-239-1 (paperback edition)

Printed in the United States of America
10  9  8  7  6  5  4  3  2  1

BOOK DESIGN BY MEIGHAN CAVANAUGH

*To my patients, whose struggles have taught me much
about the human spirit*
DR. PETER V. RABINS


*To my family*
LYNN LAUBER

# ACKNOWLEDGMENTS

The 1950s were referred to as "the age of anxiety." Fifty years later we hear much more about depression and much less about anxiety, but I continue to treat many people for complaints of nervousness and anxiety.

*Getting Old Without Getting Anxious* was written both for older individuals experiencing anxiety and for the loved ones who are supporting them. Lynn Lauber was a thoughtful, incisive writer, and I thank her for her help. Amy Goldberger, my agent, is due thanks for bringing the project to my attention and helping bring it to fruition. Janis Vallely, Lynn Lauber's agent, was also instrumental in getting the book into print.

I have chosen to dedicate this book to the many patients I have cared for over the years who have been willing to share their experiences with me. They have taught me what it is like to experience symptoms of anxiety, worry, tension, and unhappiness, and have been willing to fight the stigma of mental illness and work to their best ability in overcoming the burden of their conditions. It is our hope that others will benefit from the wisdom these individuals have brought to us.

# CONTENTS

# Part Three

# INTRODUCTION— GETTING STARTED

Growing up in Florida in the 1950s, far from my own grandparents and extended family, I sometimes adopted other people as honorary relatives.

My favorite was Mr. Louis—Uncle Lou, I called him—a longtime family friend who lived near us with his wife and daughter.

A retired geologist in his sixties, blind in one eye and arthritic, Louis was still a force of nature. Rangy and white-haired, he reminded me of a praying mantis with his long expressive hands and halting walk. I was a shy, bookish boy interested in mixing experiments in the bathroom tub, but Uncle Lou took me under his wing and urged me outside.

He trooped in front of me throughout my childhood and adolescence, pointing up at the stars and down at the rocks at my feet. He talked to me about the composition of granite; the qualities of hydrogen; the copper and tin that existed deep in veins of the earth.

From him, I have my first memories of the night sky seen through a telescope and a sense of the scientific life, in which you plumbed the world in order to discover its secrets.

His wife, Hazel, was forever hanging out the window, trying to get him to come in, put on a sweater, go to bed, but he never wanted to stop.

"Age is all in here, Peter," he told me, tapping his head.

When I got older, he was as excited as anyone to find out that I had been accepted into medical school.

"Ah, Pete . . . good for you. That's what I wanted to do myself! Now you can do it for me."

After I moved far from home in order to go to school, my visits with Uncle Lou grew more infrequent. He was in his late seventies by then, so I wasn't surprised when I noticed certain changes—forgetfulness, a remoteness, and moodiness. They were natural, I told myself, and I was so busy with my own budding life that I didn't dwell on them.

But then, after the death of Hazel, the wife he seemed to be always evading, Uncle Lou underwent a precipitous decline. The reports from home were disturbing: he'd grown so fearful that he wouldn't leave his apartment, even to go for a walk on the beach that we loved and shared so much.

When his daughter called me, she told me he'd begun seeing things.

"What do you mean?" I asked.

"They're like flashbacks. He says they're events that happened to him when he was in the war."

"What do the doctors say?"

"Just that he's senile. They don't hold out much hope."

I hadn't even realized that Uncle Lou had *been* in the war, but it turned out that there were many things about him I didn't know.

I was surprised to find out that his past had been littered with tragedies: the war, losing an infant son, losing an early inheritance to bad financial advice. He never let on to any of this during those afternoons I'd spent with him growing up. But now it was as if the past had swooped down on him.

On my infrequent visits, Uncle Lou no longer wanted to go outside for his usual, rambling walks. All his bright inquisitiveness had retreated into a blank, fearful shell. He had shut himself up, like a book, to the world.

Finally, one day, after his repeated denials of a problem, I confronted him. "Come on, Uncle Lou, something must be wrong." After much coaxing, he told me.

Not long after Hazel died, he'd been out for a walk on the dark part of the boardwalk in our hometown when he was mugged—pushed down from behind, his wallet taken. He was humiliated that he couldn't defend himself and embarrassed because he knew he shouldn't have been walking late at night by himself. Even worse, he grew preoccupied with the thought that he would get mugged again whenever he left the house. This fear had grown to the point that he couldn't shop for himself, or even go to the doctor without becoming panic-stricken.

And then the vivid nightmares began. Memories of his World War II experiences and the later death of his son began flooding his mind. He felt like a fool, and was too embarrassed and ashamed to confide in anyone.

"Promise you won't tell anyone, either, Pete."

I assumed nothing could be done to help him, and so I agreed. But I couldn't keep myself from talking about the case with some of my friends in medical school; no one seemed very interested.

"The guy's nearly eighty, right?" one student asked, and shrugged when I nodded, as if to say, *What do you expect?*

According to Uncle Lou's daughter, he declined swiftly after my last visit. I'll never forget the look on her face when I came to see him for the last time in the hospital, or her anguished question as she gripped my arm at his funeral.

"What happened to him, Peter? What could we have done?"

My desire to answer that question—one I now hear every week of my life from children of elderly sufferers of anxiety and depression—and to understand the disorder that overtook Uncle Lou's last years, not only informed my choice of geriatric psychiatry as a career but is the reason for this book.

In Lou's case, I now know he suffered from a severe case of late-onset anxiety disorder, with agoraphobic (fear of going out) and posttraumatic stress symptoms, probably triggered by the mugging but also a result of his earlier-life difficulties. These are problems that I now know could have been treated if Uncle Lou had been properly diagnosed.

I also now know that Uncle Lou was hardly alone.

It's been estimated that up to 10 percent of elderly people in this country suffer from one or another of the following common syndromes:

- Generalized anxiety disorder
- Panic disorder
- Phobia disorder
- Posttraumatic stress disorder
- Obsessive-compulsive disorder
- Depression

Uncle Lou's daughter also wasn't alone, but one of a growing number who are faced with the task of trying to help an anxious older parent.

On the basis of my twenty-five years' experience as a geriatric psychiatrist at Johns Hopkins University, I have written this book to help adult children like her assist their parents in receiving proper diagnosis, treatment, and support.

## WHY AGING MAKES US ANXIOUS

Whenever I give retirement seminars, I ask seniors what they're most worried about. And they always tell me the same things: they're anxious about losing their money, their health, and their minds.

Late life presents unique challenges that are bound to create some degree of anxiety. The older we become, the more we are all faced with a wide array of losses—from the dwindling of financial and physical independence to the death of spouses and friends. Because of this, it is not uncommon for an older parent to exhibit certain natural concerns about loss of control and physical decline.

A mother who has become recently widowed may show some nervousness about writing checks, paying bills, and handling other financial tasks that her husband took care of when he was living. A father may become fretful and anxious after moving into a retirement community from a house where he's lived for forty years. These are natural situational responses that usually diminish over time.

But an anxiety disorder isn't a natural response. It's an excessive, persistent feeling of anxiousness, depression, or distress that is not a result of a physical malady. It's a mother who is suddenly terrified to board a bus or walk to church. It's a father who begins demonstrating uncontrollable obsessive qualities, such as counting and recounting his money, or repeatedly checking that he's clean.

These symptoms interfere, even take over, a life. Yet the good news is that once a disorder has been identified and diagnosed, it can be effectively managed and treated, using a variety of proven methods and techniques tailored to an individual's specific needs.

In *Getting Old Without Getting Anxious,* I use a three-pronged approach to help:

**Inform** you of the special manifestations of anxiety in the elderly and of the ways they differ from those of the general population;

**Identify** the particular disorder your parent may be suffering from and the science of what's behind it;

**Guide** you in helping your parent fashion the best treatment options from the following modalities:

- Psychiatry and psychotherapy, including cognitive-behavioral, group, and talk therapy
- Medications, including SSRIs, benzodiazepines, buspirone, beta-blockers, tricyclics, monoamine oxidase inhibitors, and herbal alternatives, such as SAM-e, St. John's wort, and valerian
- Calming therapies, such as yoga, relaxation therapies, meditation, and tai chi
- Lifestyle enhancements such as support groups, exercise, nutrition, volunteering, creative activities, humor, and social engagement

## THE CHALLENGE OF DIAGNOSIS

Anxiety disorders can be challenging to recognize and diagnose in an elderly parent. It is not uncommon for late-life symptoms to be ignored, underestimated, or masked for the following reasons:

## ILLNESS

The frequency of chronic health problems in late life complicates diagnosis. Anxiety symptoms include such problems as difficulty breathing, a racing heart, dizziness, or forgetfulness—any of which can be a sign of a variety of illnesses from heart to lung disease. Anxiety and depression also share symptoms such as fatigue, nervousness, and sleeplessness with other physical disorders, such as thyroid dysfunction and hypoglycemia.

The fear of illness—the loss of control and independence it implies—may be one of the chief reasons some older parents are reluctant to report anxiety symptoms. The dread of Alzheimer's disease in particular can be so strong—even stronger than of death—that a parent will avoid mentioning any symptom that he fears might be associated with it.

The presence of medical illness can also camouflage an anxiety syndrome that is simultaneously present. If a parent is tackling cancer or the aftereffects of a stroke, her anxiety symptoms may remain overlooked and untreated.

One son told me, "My mother's got stage-two breast cancer—why wouldn't she be depressed?"

But the truth is that being ill doesn't necessarily mean being anxious *or* depressed, and his mother has a far better chance of handling the challenges of her disease if she isn't burdened with a clinical depression.

## MEDICATIONS

The elderly take more prescription medicines than any other age group. These medications often have side effects that cause or mimic anxiety. Drugs may also combine with each other, causing drug-drug interactions.

Seniors may also receive medications from several doctors, mix them with over-the-counter medicines and alcohol, or fail to comply with dosage instructions.

The son of one of my anxiety patients told me: "Before she came to you, my mother was taking seven different pills at once, and four of them were for anxiety. She'd gotten half of them from her doctor in Florida where she spends the winter, and the rest from her doctors in New York. She was having such weird symptoms, and nobody figured out that they were drug-related side effects. I kept saying, 'Who's keeping track of her meds?' and then it dawned on me. *No one was*. That's when I finally realized that I was going to need to take charge of some of this for her."

## FEAR

Parents may not report anxiety symptoms because they view them as signs of incompetence or mental illness; they may be afraid that they will be labeled or put away.

Some parents may have had lifelong anxiety problems that they've masked or hidden until their coping abilities become undermined by loss or trauma. A mother who was able to hide her tendency to panic when she was sheltered and protected by her husband may find herself unable to handle even an activity like food shopping, after his death.

Seniors who live alone are especially able to hide their anxiety symptoms. And in a nursing home or residential facility, staff may be unaware of a parent's normal personality and overlook signs of distress.

## ERRONEOUS ATTITUDES ABOUT AGING

Anxiety symptoms may also be dismissed or ignored in late life because they are perceived as a natural and acceptable consequence of aging.

A son brought into my office his father, who at seventy-four was suddenly suffering from vivid nightmares and flashbacks to his years as an infantry soldier in World War II. A once hearty man, he presented himself as withdrawn and fearful. Not only was he losing sleep because of these flashbacks, he had lost twenty pounds. His son, a prosperous stockbroker, was at his wits' end.

"He never would discuss this stuff when I was growing up. Now it's all he talks about," he told me. Although the son was distressed by his father's anguish, he was also fatalistic about the outcome and scoffed when I suggested cognitive-behavioral therapy. "Hey, he's not going to change at this point. If it's not physical, let's forget about it."

This is a shockingly common view—that symptoms such as these are a natural feature of late life and cannot be solved or treated. A tendency to write off the elderly and their symptoms is callous and deadly. There is no reason to consign a seventy-year-old—or a ninety-year-old—to years of needless suffering. Anxiety disorders are imminently treatable, allowing sufferers to live long lives, marked by pleasure and accomplishment, well into their eighties and beyond. I have personally encountered scores of patients who have overcome them and gone on to enjoy many vital years.

But it's not only children who view serious anxiety symptoms as a natural component of aging—often parents themselves do also.

Joe did not seek medical care for his obsessive-compulsive disorder for years, even though he later admitted that he had suffered from symptoms since he was a young man.

"I just thought I was getting old and peculiar," he told me. "I never have been one to go to the doctor. I'm not looking for trouble. You go to a doctor, you end up having an operation. Plus, I don't want anybody telling me I'm crazy."

Joe's views are not uncommon. Many older people are uncomfortable with self-disclosure or talking openly about mental health, sexual function, or other "personal" topics. They may feel a strong stigma about emotional problems or fear being called a hypochondriac.

Seniors are also more likely to have an "I can take care of it myself" attitude. Admitting that they need help and going outside the family to receive it can be a difficult thing.

Anna, a woman with agoraphobia (a fear of going out), who was from a religious family, told me, "In my family, there was a strong belief that all private troubles needed to stay inside the family circle. Talking about personal issues with outside people was viewed as airing dirty laundry and strictly forbidden." Asking for help in a family such as Anna's can even be viewed as disloyal.

In fact, there is no underestimating the fear that parents might harbor about admitting anxiety symptoms. In a time of diminishing independence, admitting to emotional problems or difficulty with mental functioning can be extremely difficult. Being aware of this, for a child, is important.

Yet once parents have the opportunity to speak freely to a nonjudgmental qualified clinician—one who can offer guidance and help—they can feel as if a great burden has been lifted.

"I had no idea that anyone else felt like I did. I suffered alone and in shame with my problem for so many years," Anna said. "I cried when my counselor told me how many other people also had this problem, and that there were treatments that could help me. Just hearing that comforted me as much as anything."

In the pages that follow I'll assist you in understanding the special ways anxiety syndromes impact your aging parent, steps you can take to have these disorders assessed and treated, and ways you can help your parent—and yourself—during these challenging times.

# PART ONE

# 1

# DIAGNOSING LATE-LIFE ANXIETY

At the beginning of the twentieth century, the average life expectancy for Americans was a little over forty years. At the start of the twenty-first, it had grown to seventy-seven. In other words, the life expectancy of the average American has nearly doubled.

That life is becoming steadily longer is definitely a happy development for seniors and the families who love them—especially when these later years are blessed with health and vigor. But there is little joy in growing older if a parent is saddled with anxiety and depression, if a mother is frightened to leave her house or a father is so isolated by phobias and panic that his days are filled with dread.

To truly benefit from the blessing of increased longevity, we need to make sure that these disorders of late life are properly recognized, diagnosed, and treated.

## NORMAL ANXIETY

Anxiety itself is not a medical problem. After bad news or a trauma, it's normal to be worried, preoccupied, and concerned. Anxiety becomes problematic when it persists long after an upsetting event, when it affects how a person functions in everyday life, or when the degree, amount, or content of the worrying seems beyond what either the person or others would perceive as "normal" or expected.

For example, I began seeing a number of older patients whose activities and travel patterns altered dramatically soon after the World Trade Center terrorist attacks. Like many people across the country, they'd canceled their travel plans, altered their usual activity patterns, and found themselves more anxious than usual.

Florence, a patient in her eighties, who'd gone to Miami for the last twenty years to stay with her sister, decided to remain in Baltimore instead. Another couple, a retired pediatrician and his wife, who'd been frequent world travelers, canceled a year's worth of cruises to remain close to home.

This skittishness to travel was a common, widespread response to the terrorist attacks. In fact, one research study that randomly sampled residents who lived in lower Manhattan, the part of the island closest to the World Trade Center, found that the number of people with anxiety symptoms nearly doubled after the attacks. Even though the majority of people did *not* experience the emergence of an anxiety state, this demonstrates how a national tragedy triggered a large dose of situational anxiety in people somewhat directly affected.[1]

Other studies showed that with the passage of time, the emotional life of most of these people returned to normal. This was also true of the patients in my office. As their fears gradually lessened, they adapted, and many began traveling as they had previously. Still, about 10 percent continued to have persistent problems and were unable to return to the way they had been before. For this group, the terrorist attacks triggered anxiety syndromes that they may have harbored all along.

So why is it that one person will be resilient in the face of these kinds of events while another will be seriously affected?

It turns out that certain elements add to the risk of developing an anxiety disorder. They include:

**Proximity to an upsetting or traumatic event.** On September 11, a person was at greater risk if he lived on Canal Street in lower Manhattan than if he lived farther away—in Harlem, for example.

**Temperament.** A person who has responded to stressors earlier in life by worrying excessively is more likely to experience persistent worry after a traumatic event. In other words, the personality trait "tendency to worry" describes not only a person's usual level of anxiety, but also predicts whether he will become emotionally overwhelmed by anxiety in the face of a major stressor.

**A family history of anxiety.** There is evidence from a number of research studies that the tendency to worry is partly inherited. This is best demonstrated in studies of identical twins who were adopted out and raised by different families—often twins who had no contact with each other. These studies show that the tendency to worry is partly predicted by the level of worry in the genetic parents, *as well as* in the adoptive parents. In other words, genetics plays a role, and so does environment.

**Early-life trauma or being subject to a stressful event early in life.** A number of studies have suggested that individuals who report significant physical or psychological trauma as children are more likely to report having anxiety and depression as adults.

Putting these risks into perspective means that even someone who was anxious as a child, had a nervous father who deserted the family, and lived near the site of a disaster will not *necessarily* develop an anxiety problem, but has an increased likelihood due to these elements.

Late life adds another layer of stressors to the mix. The elderly are much more likely than the young to be experiencing physical illnesses, suffering the loss of friends or loved ones, moving to a new environment, or undergoing a change in status. Each of these adds an extra burden and increases the likelihood for development of an anxiety disorder.

One of my patients, Frieda, was moved out of her family home into her son's duplex apartment, receiving rehab after a stroke, and dealing with the death of her husband—all in the space of a year. In her case, a lifelong battle with panic resurfaced and grew even more severe.

# THE DETECTIVE WORK OF DIAGNOSIS

When an elderly patient comes into my office displaying anxiety symptoms, I often have to do a bit of detective work to discover the root of the problem. So many seniors are on medication, suffering from physical ailments, or reluctant to admit emotional distress that diagnosis isn't always simple. Besides, each older patient is a walking catalogue of life experiences so varied that each presentation of symptoms is unique. That's why it can be so challenging for a clinician—let alone an adult child—to recognize when there's a problem, let alone pinpoint the specific disorder.

Special issues that complicate diagnosis in later life include:

## LACK OF A PSYCHOLOGICAL VOCABULARY

Older parents are often uncomfortable with introspection and may identify the presence of emotional problems and mental-health issues with stigma and shame, as evidence of moral or physical weakness. They may be uneasy talking openly about mental health, sexual function, and other "embarrassing" or personal topics. "Depression" and "Alzheimer's" are especially dreaded words.

Lacking a psychological vocabulary, seniors with anxiety may describe physical complaints that they feel more comfortable discussing. Instead of reporting anxiety or depression, for example, they may talk about general body aches and pains, fatigue, restlessness, lack of appetite, or insomnia.

Cecil, a patient of mine, complained of persistent facial tightness, especially in his jaw, and headaches. It turned out that since the illness and recent death of his wife, he'd grown so tense and anxious that he'd been grinding his teeth at night. He was able to report the headaches, but it was not as easy for him to talk about the anxiety and pain related to losing his wife.

## VIEWING DOCTORS AS GODS

Many older-generation parents view doctors as venerated figures with whom they are reluctant to discuss emotional problems. They may also fear being labeled hypochondriacs, view regular checkups as excessive and un-warranted, or feel that they don't want to waste a doctor's time.

Or they may simply fear a doctor's diagnosis.

As my patient Marion told me, "If I complain about the fact that I'm getting anxious, my doctor might tell my kids that it's time for me to give up my apartment and move into assisted living. I'm not ready for that."

## OLDER-MALE SYNDROME

In a culture that encourages males to be rugged and self-sufficient, it can be especially tough for them to admit that they're anxious or depressed. Asking a doctor for help goes against the masculine ethos many older men grew up with, which puts a premium on autonomy and strength.

Undoubtedly, this was part of Cecil's reluctance to admit his anxiety to me. A veteran police officer, he finally confessed that he equated being sad and upset with being weak and needy.

## DIFFERENTIATING THE PHYSICAL FROM THE PSYCHOLOGICAL

The high rate of chronic illness and medication use in late life makes separating the medical and psychological causes of anxiety symptoms especially challenging. Some illnesses, such as cardiac and lung problems, produce symptoms that are similar to those of classic anxiety disorders—erratic heartbeat, shortness of breath, and difficulty breathing. This issue is also complicated by the frequency of Alzheimer's disease or dementia in late life, since anxiety symptoms may also be a part of these disorders.

A patient named Hal told me: "After I had my heart attack, nobody noticed that I was also depressed. Everything was centered on my heart and how my valves and arteries were functioning. When I didn't want to eat or see anyone, they just blamed it all on my cardiac problems. It took my son making an appointment with a therapist before anyone took notice."

## HIGH FREQUENCY OF SITUATIONAL PROBLEMS IN LATE LIFE

Older people are faced with such a wide variety of losses and changes—from the death of spouses and friends to relocation and retirement—that the likelihood is very high that they will suffer from quite natural phases of transitory or passing anxiety. These anxieties, while serious, usually are not long-lasting and typically do not interfere with a parent's life. But their reality must be taken into account during diagnosis and distinguished from persistent, severe, disabling anxiety that requires clinical intervention.

"Some friends said it was normal for me to be scared to leave the apartment after my husband died," a patient named Mary said. "But as the months passed, I kept thinking: Shouldn't I be getting over this by now? Shouldn't I be feeling better instead of worse? When I was still isolated and anxious after six months, my granddaughter finally talked me into seeing a doctor."

# HOW TO DISTINGUISH A DISORDER FROM NATURAL ANXIETY

Since anxiety is so common, distinguishing between a parent who is undergoing expected and normal responses to the changes aging has brought into his life from one who is feeling tense and anxious for no clear reason becomes one of the most important aspects of the diagnostic evaluation.

Just how tense *should* a man be who's recently lost his wife? How nervous *should* a parent be who is facing chemotherapy or has diminished mobility because of a stroke? Being at least somewhat anxious in the face of these events is normal; in fact, being unmoved by such events would be a sign in itself that something is amiss.

Given the many challenges older parents face, how can you tell when a parent is having anxiety that is appropriate or troublesome enough to be checked out by a doctor?

## 3 WARNING SIGNS THAT SYMPTOMS MIGHT SIGNAL AN ANXIETY DISORDER

If symptoms are:

### 1. Persistent

The chronic nature of symptoms distinguishes normal anxiety from anxiety disorders. For example, it is natural for an older father to experience aftereffects from a car accident. He may be nervous about driving, avoid the area of the accident, even have nightmares about it. But if he persists in reliving the accident, refuses to drive over time, and remains preoccupied by his experience after three months, his symptoms may signal a disorder.

### 2. Excessive

With anxiety syndromes, everyday activities become suddenly overwhelming. What was previously an annual visit to the doctor can become a dreaded and panicked trip. A child's vacation is the occasion for anguished rumination about the likelihood of a plane crash. A trip to the grocery store cannot be managed without constant checking of locks or panic about entering a crowded place.

Such intrusive worry and overreaction cannot be reasoned away. Even when a patient realizes that such thoughts are foolish, silly, or irrational, he cannot stop them through willpower alone.

### 3. Life-altering

A change in a parent's everyday functioning is a warning sign of an anxiety or depressive disorder. Alterations in eating habits, sleep patterns, and a lack of interest in activities a person once enjoyed are important signs that shouldn't be overlooked. Of course, they can also signal the development of a new medical problem, so a thorough medical assessment is essential.

It's natural for a woman to fall under a spell of grief and become withdrawn after the death of her spouse. But when a woman who was previously sociable and outgoing remains tense, morose, or secluded for several months, you should be concerned that an anxiety or depressive disorder has developed.

## LOOKING FOR PATTERNS

One of my main tasks when assessing a new patient is to look for a pattern of symptoms.

Mrs. Gordon was brought into my office by her daughter, who'd made an appointment because of concern that her mother was becoming increasingly forgetful and anxious about becoming ill. Mrs. Gordon sat on the sidelines, twisting a tissue, as her daughter, a lawyer who lived in another state, detailed the problems. Mrs. Gordon had locked herself out of her apartment several times, lost her billfold, and wasn't sleeping. When the daughter arrived for a visit, she found her mother still in bed in the middle of the afternoon, and her apartment in shambles.

"My mother is a neatness freak, so I know she must be losing it," the daughter said. "My friend's mother has Alzheimer's, and this is exactly how it started. I want to get her on medication now, before she gets worse."

Mrs. Gordon seemed intimidated by her high-powered daughter who emanated impatience and disapproval. It was clear that the daughter had already diagnosed her mother's condition and wanted it handled as swiftly as a piece of litigation. I wasn't so sure I was seeing the full picture, so I spoke with her internist, ordered a full battery of physical tests, and asked mother and daughter to return the next week.

On the second visit, I asked the daughter to remain in the waiting room while I talked to her mother. Mrs. Gordon visibly relaxed when I assured her that her tests were all in normal range and began asking her searching questions.

She reported that, at her daughter's urging, she had recently moved out of the house where she had lived most of her life into an assisted-living apartment nearer her daughter's home. This was a terribly disorienting experience for her. She was now miles away from a close-knit neighborhood where she had lived since she was a girl, and she could no longer easily visit her friends. Since she'd begun spending so much of her time alone, she'd developed a number of symptoms that worried her, including an erratic heartbeat.

Her daughter, however, expected her to quickly adjust to this new environment. Mrs. Gordon told me: "She has no patience with me when I tell her I'm nervous or I'm worried about my heart." She complained to me of feeling overwhelmingly tense, anxious, and guilty.

Though they ebb and flow, anxiety disorders are often lifelong in duration. Even when a current episode of distress is linked to a specific trauma, a parent or family member may remember other earlier episodes that seemed to arise out of the blue. Indeed, as we talked, Mrs. Gordon admitted that she'd experienced similar symptoms—insomnia, forgetfulness, overworry—a number of times in her life, but had kept these problems to herself.

While anxiety symptoms are often associated with a number of dementias, the more I listened to Mrs. Gordon the more I suspected Alzheimer's wasn't her problem. When I looked at her responses to the Hamilton Anxiety Scale (see page 27), her performance on an in-office cognitive test, her normal medical test results, and her self-reported past history of anxiety, I was sure that she was suffering from generalized anxiety disorder and depression, not Alzheimer's.

Sometimes we think we know our parents so well that we don't pay close attention to what they're telling us, and we may be surprised by our blind spots and misperceptions. It's important to listen closely to what a parent says when reporting anxiety symptoms. Besides helping in the eventual diagnosis, closely attending to an elderly parent's feelings and complaints can be therapeutic in itself.

## STEPS IN EVALUATION

A medical evaluation is always an essential first component in diagnosing anxiety. It is only after medical problems or illnesses are ruled out that anxiety symptoms can be fully evaluated.

This is because a number of medical illnesses—thyroid overactivity (hyperthyroidism), hypoglycemia, cardiac and pulmonary problems, to name a few—can actually mimic anxiety or produce anxiety-like symptoms.

A medical history generally covers the current symptoms, family history of medical, neurologic, and psychiatric illness, past and present alcohol use, injuries, prior hospitalizations, operations, and allergies. It should also include a patient's current medicines, both prescription and over the counter, since certain drugs and drug-drug interactions can cause nervousness.

Diagnostic workups should include blood tests that look at red and white blood-cell count, hormone levels, thyroid function, and electrolytes. Other standard tests that may be performed include liver and kidney function tests and an electrocardiogram.

A psychological history is also essential, as well as an analysis of cognitive and perceptual abilities. Anxiety rating scales, such as the Hamilton Anxiety Scale, or self-rated scales, such as the Beck Anxiety Inventory, may be helpful.

Tests that are utilized to evaluate memory and thinking include:

■ Giving a parent a list of three or four words, then asking him to recall the words three minutes later.

■ Asking a parent the date. Although some people might be off a day or two, most without cognitive impairment will be close.

■ Asking the person to draw a picture of a clock, to write in the numbers, then to write in a specific time—say, ten minutes past eleven. This is an exercise that most people with dementia or Alzheimer's disease are unable to do.

After the physical exam and laboratory evaluation have ruled out physical ailments, I ask my patients the following questions or have them fill out an anxiety-rating scale.

## COMMON PSYCHOLOGICAL ASSESSMENT QUESTIONS

Do you consider yourself to be anxious?

When did your anxiety start?

Have there been any major changes in your life?

Do you have any physical symptoms related to your anxiety?

In what order did these symptoms occur?

Are you aware of an event that may have triggered these anxiety symptoms?

What impact have they had on your life?

Have they interfered with your daily functioning? If so, how?

Is there anyone else in your family who suffers from similar symptoms?

Is there anything that improves your anxiety?

Is there anything that makes your anxiety worse?

## OTHER SCREENING QUESTIONS DESIGNED TO PINPOINT SPECIFIC DISORDERS

Do you find yourself terrified to leave the house or to be in public? (*for social disorder*)

Do you check things repeatedly or wash your hands over and over? (*for obsessive-compulsive disorder*)

Do you feel an overwhelming fear of a particular object or situation, such as getting on an elevator? (*for phobia disorder*)

Do you ever find yourself overly preoccupied with an early trauma in your life? (*for posttraumatic stress disorder*)

Do you feel yourself to be generally worried all the time? (*for generalized anxiety disorder*)

Do you ever suffer from overwhelming feelings of panic? (*for panic disorder*)

In my experience, once a disorder is diagnosed and I've had a chance to explain it to a patient, as well as to highlight possible treatments, at least some of my patient's anxiety is relieved.

Jerome, who had suffered most of his life from a phobic disorder that he experienced primarily as claustrophobia (fear of closed spaces such as elevators or closets), told me: "I was embarrassed all my life by my limitations and always felt apologetic and guilty when it interfered with activities my family wanted to do. When I heard that there was a name for it, and that there was treatment that could potentially help me, I finally stopped blaming myself."

## CREATIVE DIAGNOSIS AND TREATMENT

An older patient, such as Tom T., provides a number of diagnostic challenges.

A seventy-five-year-old salesman and World War II vet, Tom had grown increasingly morose with age, and had developed memory loss after open-heart surgery. Formerly a garrulous, outgoing man, he had become listless, antisocial, and had begun lashing out at his wife in fights that were becoming frightening in their intensity. As far as his wife and children were concerned, Tom was clearly depressed, but he would not admit to any sadness or psychological problems; the most he'd say was that he felt irritable much of the time. He was part of the World War II generation who thought any such admission meant he was soft or weak.

"He's always perfectly charming whenever we go to the doctor. He always says everything's great," his wife reported. "Then we get back home and start fighting again."

Since Tom was adamant in his refusal to discuss any sort of problem with his long-term primary-care doctor, his wife was growing desperate. Then one afternoon, when she was having a checkup of her own, she began talking to the nurse practitioner and broke down in tears. "The nurse really listened to me," she later admitted. "She told me to bring Tom in on another pretext, getting a flu shot, and that she would talk to him."

The nurse practitioner was able to talk to Tom in a nonthreatening, empathic way. After his medical tests were found to be normal, she told him:

"I don't know about you, but my husband gets moody sometimes, just like your wife says you do. Would you be willing to try this pill he takes and see if it helps you as much as it helps him?"

This approach worked. Tom agreed to try Zoloft and, within six weeks, his wife reported that his dark moods had greatly diminished.

"The difference this has made in our daily lives is enormous," she reported. "I'm so grateful to the nurse for managing to talk to Tom without even bringing up the word 'depression,' which would have closed down his doors. I can't think of any other way he would have agreed to try an antidepressant."

My own research suggests that older patients like Tom, who suffer from major depression, are less likely to report feelings of sadness than younger people; even though they may have all the other symptoms—such as trouble sleeping, low energy, and appetite loss.

Tom's case illustrates how creative methods can often make all the difference in diagnosis and treatment. It also shows how clinicians other than doctors can be helpful in dealing with an anxious older patient. While it's important for a person who develops symptoms to have a thorough medical workup, preferably by a primary-care doctor, some patients may not have a physician with whom they're comfortable. Because of this, social workers, nurse practitioners, and psychologists may be the clinicians whom elderly patients first see with their anxiety symptoms.

This is also true in long-term facilities and managed-care environments, where patients are more likely to reveal anxiety symptoms to nurses, social workers, and psychologists than to doctors. Furthermore, research suggests that primary-care practitioners, who are often the first-line responders for mental disorders, are not as well informed as mental-health professionals about depression and anxiety disorders, and are therefore more likely to undertreat them.[2]

In the end, a partnership of cooperation and communication between family, clinicians, physicians, and the patient leads to the highest quality care and the best treatment results.

## CONSIDERATIONS WHEN CHOOSING A CLINICIAN

Has the clinician received specialized training in geriatrics?

Is he/she communicative, friendly, and easy to understand?

Does the clinician encourage family participation and treat the patient with respect?

Will the clinician accept supplemental insurance or Medicare?

Is he/she willing to follow up on treatment?

Does the clinician adequately explain medications, side effects, and plan to monitor use?

How far is the clinician's office from where the patient lives?

Will he/she agree to make home visits or be available after hours?

# Hamilton Anxiety Scale[3]

## I. SYMPTOM RATING SCALE (0 = NOT PRESENT, 4 = DISABLING)

**A. ANXIOUS MOOD**
1. Worries
2. Anticipates worst

**B. TENSION**
1. Startles
2. Cries easily
3. Restless
4. Trembling

**C. FEARS**
1. Fear of the dark
2. Fear of strangers
3. Fear of being alone
4. Fear of animals

**D. INSOMNIA**
1. Difficulty falling asleep or staying asleep
2. Difficulty with nightmares

**E. INTELLECTUAL**
1. Poor concentration
2. Memory impairment

**F. DEPRESSED MOOD**
1. Decreased interest in activities
2. Anhedonia
3. Insomnia

**G. SOMATIC COMPLAINTS: MUSCULAR**
1. Muscle aches or pains
2. Bruxism

**H. SOMATIC COMPLAINTS: SENSORY**
1. Tinnitus
2. Blurred vision

**I. CARDIOVASCULAR SYMPTOMS**
1. Tachycardia
2. Palpitations
3. Chest pain
4. Sensation of feeling faint

**J. RESPIRATORY SYMPTOMS**
1. Chest pressure
2. Choking sensation
3. Shortness of breath

**K. GASTROINTESTINAL SYMPTOMS**
1. Dysphagia
2. Nausea or vomiting
3. Constipation
4. Weight loss
5. Abdominal fullness

**L. GENITOURINARY SYMPTOMS**
1. Urinary frequency or urgency
2. Dysmenorrhea
3. Impotence

**M. AUTONOMIC SYMPTOMS**
1. Dry mouth
2. Flushing
3. Pallor
4. Sweating

*(continued)*

## Hamilton Anxiety Scale

### I. SYMPTOM RATING SCALE (0 = NOT PRESENT, 4 = DISABLING)

**N. BEHAVIOR AT INTERVIEW**
1. Fidgets
2. Tremor
3. Paces

### II. INTERPRETATION

**A. ABOVE 14 SYMPTOMS ARE GRADED ON SCALE**
1. Not present: 0
2. Very severe symptoms: 4

**B. CRITERIA**
1. Mild anxiety (minimum for anxiolytic): 18
2. Moderate anxiety: 25
3. Severe anxiety: 30

# 2

# BEHIND THE SYMPTOMS: UNDERSTANDING THE CAUSES OF ANXIETY DISORDERS

A teacher named Carla was telling me about her father, William. "My dad has panic attacks and suffers from PTSD [posttraumatic stress disorder] related to his combat experience during World War II. Ever since there have been terrorism alerts, his symptoms have been even worse. He has spells when he feels like he can't breathe or leave the house. He's put duct tape around the windows and plastic sheeting over the screen doors. Whenever the alert goes higher, he calls and wants me to keep the kids home from school. I know this is a disorder, but my coworkers are nervous and buying duct tape, too. What makes my father's response so much more extreme?"

In anxious times, people of all ages feel jittery. There's so much to worry about—from terrorism, to job instabilities, to war. Worry and anxiety are appropriate, healthy responses to stressful times and situations. When people are in danger or under threat, their brains release hormones that prepare them to fight or flee. To prepare the body for action, the heartbeat quickens and the muscles tense; vision and hearing become more acute and focused. These reactions typically go away once a person no longer feels threatened. But when a susceptible person such as Carla's father is faced with too much anxiety or fear, these appropriate physical states take on a life of their own and extend far beyond a few sleepless nights or days of uneasiness. The persistence and debilitating nature of these symptoms are what constitute a disorder.

But where do individual differences come from?

Why is Carla's father debilitated by stress that leaves so many others, faced with similar circumstances, only mildly or transiently anxious?

## COMPLEX THREADS

There is a complex, invisible reaction occurring inside Carla's anxious father when he's in the throes of his anxiety. Syndromes such as his are the result of an interweaving of biology, learning, environment, and temperament, strands that are not easy to separate or unravel. But neuroimaging technologies that allow us to peek into the living brain, genetic studies that locate chromosomal areas implicated in the formation of depression and other disorders, and research on the impact of early life experiences can help us understand more clearly than ever some of the underlying causes.

But why does it matter what is actually going on in a parent when he's having an anxiety attack?

Why is it significant that a sophisticated brain scan of a patient with obsessive-compulsive disorder (OCD) highlights increased activity in certain brain structures that diminishes once she's been treated?

What are the ramifications of a wide range of studies suggesting that a person is more likely to suffer from panic if a close family member does also? Or other research suggesting that anxiety sufferers have an oversensitivity of the brain receptors for the chemical neurotransmitters norepinephrine (a form of adrenaline), serotonin, and GABA (gamma aminobutyric acid)?

How does it help us to know that early trauma or abuse not only causes enduring psychological scars, but actually induces permanent changes in the brain?

There are a number of reasons why it's important to understand the underlying role that biologic abnormalities, genetic predispositions, and life experience play in your parent's anxiety disorder. Such understanding:

### ■ Increases empathy and understanding

Realizing that your panicked mother is undergoing a physiological experience that's causing adrenaline and other stress hormones to flood her body can increase your awareness and allow you to be more supportive.

"My father's rituals ruled his life, and mine," a son of an OCD sufferer told me. "They were completely nonsensical, as far as I was concerned. I was always losing patience with him when he stopped to count the bricks on the side of the building or the number of times that two appeared in the newspaper article he was reading. He exhausted and exasperated me for years. Then his doc put him on medication and therapy, and he changed—I mean *really* changed. All of a sudden he seemed nearly normal, for the first time I could remember. And it hit me—if medication helped him, then there was some serious malfunction he'd been saddled with all those years. I found it sobering that I'd never quite realized this."

Appreciating the biological and psychological basis underlying a disorder can help you realize that a parent is vulnerable, because of genetic or experiential factors, not a weakling or a malingerer.

One daughter told me: "I realized I was being far less sympathetic to my phobic mother than to my father, who was suffering similar symptoms because of dementia. When our doctor explained to me about brain neurochemicals and how my mother's tests suggested hers may be out of balance, it gave me new insight."

### ■ Identifies the need for treatment

Understanding the basis of fear and anxiety and how they affect different areas of the brain makes it easier to match treatments to an individual's needs. Just as these disorders often have unique and complex causes, so the treatments can be tailored for each patient, personalized from the best mix of the various options available.

Locating the underlying mechanisms of anxiety symptoms can provide clues to how they can be manipulated and eradicated. For example, if brain circuits normally involved in fear and anxiety begin functioning in a way that's destructive, it's possible they can be "fixed" with either medication or cognitive-behavior therapy.

In one study, patients with particular patterns of brain activity were found to respond well to Paxil for OCD and depression. Sophisticated brain imagery scans called PET (positron-emission tomography) scans, taken before and after treatment, showed that the individuals whose OCD symptoms improved had higher pretreatment activity in certain areas of the brain.

Such studies may revolutionize the ways in which depression patients are treated. They may help minimize the use of drugs on patients who are unlikely to positively respond, cutting down on expensive, time-consuming trial and error. They can also help clinicians tailor unique treatment plans, geared for individual patients.[1]

### ■ Changes the sufferer's perception

The guilt, fear, shame, and misunderstanding that accompany anxiety disorders are a burden under which many older patients suffer.

Many seniors have a "pioneer" mentality toward emotional problems, believing that they should be able to tough them out on their own because their disorders aren't serious enough to warrant treatment. Admitting that they need help and talking about emotional issues outside of their families can be extremely difficult.

Understanding the basis of a disorder can be a major part of treatment and healing. "I don't feel such shame since the doctor explained to me that I probably inherited this from my family, and that it might involve some kind of chemical malfunction in my brain," one father, a devoutly religious man who had suffered from clinical depression most of his life, told me. "I was always going to confession, thinking that I'd done something to deserve this terrible feeling of doom. Now I realize it wasn't my fault."

### ■ Helps sufferers accept treatment and stick with it

Knowledge and education about the underlying causes of a disorder can be a powerful and liberating tool for older patients, one that may help them view treatment in a new light.

"I figured I went to physical therapy when my knee was injured, so why not therapy for my mind?" an elderly mother told me.

Your parent is also more likely to stick to a treatment when it's rooted in an understanding of the disorder and the possible reasons behind it.

"When my doctor explained that my brain had been 'traumatized' during my years of combat, and that I needed help to change my thinking and behavior, I finally could accept it," a posttraumatic-stress patient said. "Before that, doctors treated me like I was crazy or weak, and I always stopped going. But now that I feel I understand what happened to me, I'm more motivated to help myself."

## THE BIOLOGY OF ANXIETY

Stress and anxiety are not only part of modern life, they're essential for our survival. Because of the natural warning system hardwired in us, we're able to calculate that a menacing look on a stranger's face signals danger and we should cross the road, or that a weaving car is being driven erratically and we need to change lanes.

We all require a certain amount of anxiety to make it in the modern world. Your parent needs a healthy dose in order to survive. Without anxiety, your mother might take a walk around her neighborhood in the middle of the night, or your father might reach out to pet a dog that is about to attack him.

In the face of danger, our bodies experience physiological changes, involving heart rate, abdominal discomfort, blood flow, and breathing. But with an anxiety disorder, these same changes are triggered inappropriately in situations that do not warrant them. Brain sensors that make a person attuned to danger malfunction and make him overly sensitive.

A mother may find herself responding to a trip to the drugstore as if she were facing some calamitous natural disaster, with dizziness, a pounding heart, and sweating. The backfiring of a car can throw a father with PTSD into a time warp, so that he reexperiences a mortar attack from decades before.

The amygdala is the ancient part of the brain that serves as fear central not only in humans, but in many living organisms, from alligators to chimpanzees. The amygdala is an almond-shaped grouping of neurons or nerve cells deep in the temporal lobe of the brain. (The word *amygdala* means "almond" in Latin.) This small area is amazingly powerful, because it controls the development of emotional memory and acts as a clearinghouse for the integration of stimuli that provoke fear. As part of our first response system, it sets off powerful signals to let us know that we're in dangerous or threatening situations.

At the sight of a gun in an attacker's hand, the amygdala in effect cries "Watch out!" and produces signals that release stress hormones such as cortisol and adrenaline, which cause a pounding heart, muscle contraction, sweating, and dilated pupils, as well as increase the breathing rate and prepare muscle to operate maximally. These hormones also heighten the awareness of external surroundings and improve vision (by dilation of the pupils) and hearing. And all of this happens involuntarily, unconsciously, within moments of the sight of a gun.

We want our amygdala to react this way, with heightened, focused attention. We want to be able to think quickly in an emergency. If a car is swerving in front of us or an enemy soldier is nearby, our survival depends upon our paying instant attention and ignoring less important distractions. We'd be in trouble if our bodies made us stop and consider each movement—"Now I have to move this leg; now I have to focus my vision"—or if we were distracted by a toothache or a buzzing insect. The amygdala is the part of the brain that allows us this swift, exclusive reaction. In fact, natural selection may have favored those of us who are most attuned to stress and anxiety—we are the ones who reacted successfully in dangerous situations and survived.

The amygdala is also the part of the brain that says "Remember this!" whenever we've had an emotional or traumatic experience. As such, it is also a part of the memory system and helps us learn about dangerous situations and either avoid them or be prepared for them in the future.

Some research theorizes that traumatic events leave deeply etched "fear memories" or emotional imprints in the amygdala and that it's these memories that trigger anxiety disorders if they become inadvertently or improperly "recalled."

Research with rats indicates that once a fear is learned, brain pathways form that make it possible to learn future fears more quickly.[2] We're not born with a fear of rottweilers, for example, but can readily learn to fear them if provided with a negative experience.

The average person bitten by a rottweiler is likely to feel fear even more rapidly the next time he's confronted with one, but this fear will typically fade if the dog is encountered several times without incident. Yet for someone with an anxiety disorder, the amygdala has learned the fear far *too* well. Instead of the reaction being suppressed in the future, it actually becomes more likely to occur. After a rottweiler bite, a phobic person might develop a fear of all dogs or develop agoraphobia and become fearful of leaving the house. A PTSD sufferer might experience a fear response—a pounding heart and rapid breathing—at the mere memory of his previous attack.

Most often the sufferer isn't even aware what an anxiety trigger is; he simply hears or sees something, and a cascading series of events begins in his body. Noise, a sudden movement, or simply the circumstances of ordinary life can activate the process. The person's brain is sensing a threat, though he can't say why. It's as if the body has observed something that never made it to the conscious brain, but was sent directly to the amygdala.

Certainly stress has a protective function; keeping us wary of frightening strangers, dark alleys, and recklessly speeding cars. We know that we'd be in trouble without a well-functioning amygdala. For example, researchers studying a young woman who suffered brain damage in this area found her to be socially inappropriate with strangers, overly trusting and easily taken advantage of. They hypothesized that the damage to the woman's brain had erased the protective function of the amygdala, along with her notion of fear.[3]

This line of reasoning is supported by other studies showing that those with a damaged amygdala cannot experience threatening faces as unfriendly or recognize fear in someone else's face, responses that are almost instantaneous and automatic in a person with a normally functioning brain.

While this hardwired wariness is essential, it's not beneficial for the body—especially the aging body—to be soaked in a constant bath of anxiety and stress. A panic sufferer's chronic worry about another attack may trigger other physical illness, such as heart problems and irritable bowel syndrome, and increase the likelihood of major depression. A patient with generalized anxiety disorder (GAD) is a veritable worry factory, oversensitive to her environment and drenching her body with daily doses of cortisol, norepinephrine, and GABA. The chronic stress can affect immunity and make people more vulnerable to infection and disease.

These symptoms are also a devastating added burden on an aging parent already coping with the challenges of growing older. The feelings of hopelessness and helplessness these disorders engender can lead to deepening symptoms, depression, and a withdrawal from life. That's why it is so essential that late-life anxiety disorders be diagnosed and treated.

## IN THE GENES

It's been well established through a wide variety of family, adoption, and twin studies that anxiety disorders have a genetic component.

This means that if your parent is suffering from OCD or phobia or depression, you may be at a higher risk of developing the disorder yourself. Almost half of panic sufferers, for example, have at least one relative who is also affected.[4] This doesn't mean you will *necessarily* develop the same disorder that a parent or sibling is suffering from, only that your risk is increased.

Genetics may explain why some people exposed to traumatic events develop anxiety disorders while others remain unfazed. In fact, research has shown that one or more fearful experiences can trigger a genetically susceptible person to respond in an excessive way to situations where others would experience either little or no fear and anxiety.

Studies have indicated that individuals who have inherited particular variations in a gene involved in transporting serotonin into brain cells experience more activity in the amygdala—in other words, more fear. This could either predispose them to develop anxiety disorders or make them more vigilant—depending upon other factors, including life experience and environment.[5]

What this indicates is that some individuals *have a greater tendency* to react to potentially or actually threatening situations with a heightened response. Because it does not appear to mean that predisposed individuals *inevitably* will respond in this way, there are presumably other genetic or learned factors that can protect against or lessen the tendency. If this research bears fruit, we might soon be able to identify vulnerable individuals and teach them techniques that lower their risk of developing a disorder in the future, even in the face of the inevitable stresses of life.

Similar exciting findings might apply to other conditions. A large group of U.S. researchers recently completed the first survey of the entire human genome and discovered a number of chromosomal regions that may contain the genetic keys to susceptibility to depression, schizophrenia, and addictions.

Studies of twins have long demonstrated that genetic factors account for half or more of the risk for developing major depression, but locating those genes has proven difficult, since a number of genes are involved, and only people with certain combinations develop the disorder.

This survey found nineteen loci (small regions on chromosomes where genes reside) that seem to influence susceptibility to depressive disorders, as well as a small chromosome region that affects the vulnerability of women to depression. This is of interest, since women are twice as likely as men to develop this disorder, and genetic differences can now be shown to account for at least a portion of that increased risk. Another group found that one of these regions might be contributing to the development of both depression and panic.[6]

Why are such studies relevant? Because the identification of susceptible genes can lead to development of more effective medicines targeted to treat depression in specific individuals. It might also provide new insight into disease prevention and help clinicians match patients with treatments suited to their unique needs.

The durability of inherited characteristics can be seen in the case of Maryanne and her daughter Nancy, who were separated for thirty-five years. As a young, unwed mother, Maryanne had given up her daughter for adoption, believing that her child would have a better chance in a more educated, well-adjusted environment than her own working-class home. Her father was a moody, taciturn alcoholic, and her mother suffered from manic-depressive illness, also called bipolar disorder, and rarely left the house. Maryanne herself had suffered from bouts of depression since girlhood. "I was sure my daughter would have a better life with a healthier, more adjusted family," she said.

The baby was placed with a wealthy professional family in another state. The father was a neurologist, the mother a retired nurse; there were three other siblings, all boys. They were an outgoing, sports-loving, gregarious family, but Nancy never quite felt she belonged.

"Even before I knew I was adopted, I felt that I didn't fit in. I was shy and moody a lot of the time. My brothers were constantly telling me that I didn't know how to have fun. I was always wondering if there was something wrong with me."

When Nancy married and became pregnant in her thirties, she got interested in finding her biological family. "Once I became pregnant, it really obsessed me. I wanted to know whose genes I was passing on."

Maryanne was in her sixties and on medication for depression when Nancy contacted her after discovering that her birth father had died long ago.

"It was such a relief to meet her; I was absolutely amazed by how alike we are," Nancy said. "Her voice sounds like mine; our bone structure is very similar; she even holds her arms the same way I do. But even more important, she has my same temperament. She's shy in crowds; she's moody and standoffish. In the middle of my happy-go-lucky family, I always stuck out like a sore thumb. Now I understand where it comes from!"

For her part, being reunited with her long-lost daughter changed the way Maryanne viewed the world. "I was always such a sad sack, especially after the adoption. I never wanted to have another child; I just kind of retreated from the world and turned into an old lady. But seeing Nancy—and now my granddaughter—has made me so much more hopeful and happy."

People look for simple explanations for complex events. A daughter wants to blame her mother's panic on the fact that she was in the vicinity of the Oklahoma City bombing; a nurse wants to explain away her father's nervousness by brain chemistry alone.

Yet the story of Maryanne and Nancy illustrates the way that both genetics *and* experience impact our temperaments and view of life in complex ways that scientists and clinicians are just now beginning to understand.

## ENVIRONMENT AND EXPERIENCE

Even if we are predisposed by our genetic makeup to develop an anxiety disorder, we are more than our circuitry, DNA, and shifting levels of neurochemicals. The brain is not static but molded by the events and experiences of life. The landscape you are born into and interact with; whether you're a man or a woman, raised in a loving or violent family environment; whether your past has been relatively trauma-free or you've suffered abuses or been witness to terrible atrocities—all these play a part in how the brain develops and how we experience the world.

We know experience affects the biology of the brain and vice versa. Studies by the National Institute of Mental Health suggest that those who suffer one or more highly traumatic life events have triple the risk of the average population of developing GAD, as well as exhibiting the kinds of changes on brain scans that indicate their brains have been altered.

We also know that what may be a precipitating trigger in one person may barely affect another. PTSD is a disorder that, by its very definition, is precipitated by a traumatic life experience, such as being near the World Trade Center on the morning of 9/11. The complexity arrives from the fact that not everyone who was near the World Trade Center developed PTSD symptoms. Those who did may have had prior life experience that predisposed them, as well as a biological propensity.

Research has shown that environment not only has a major effect on our neural circuitry, but that experience actually causes structural changes in the brain.[7] The brain's "plasticity" has been demonstrated by such neuroscientists as Nobel Prize winner Dr. Eric Kandel of Columbia University. It is still a mystery exactly how past and present environments shape circuitry that connects emotions with pathways that release neurochemicals. But one thing is for certain—we are not simply hostages of our DNA.

## THE STAGES OF LIFE

What happens to us in childhood has a profound effect on our development and on whether we are likely to suffer anxiety disorders later in life. There's evidence that patterns of emotional responsiveness are developed in childhood and young adulthood. People who are raised in threatening or unpredictable circumstances have an increased likelihood of emotional instability or over- or underreaction to a stress. For example, individuals brought up during World War II in areas where there was deprivation and starvation have, as a group, more emotional problems in adulthood than those who were raised in an environment of stable prosperity.

There are also certain stages of human life when development occurs biologically and experientially. When they happen at the wrong time or degree, or they're marked by trauma or extreme stress, they can have long-term effects.

Many theorists have suggested that human development must unfold in a certain sequence for a person to be psychologically robust. For example, psychologist Erik Erikson described a theory of human development that consists of eight crucial steps that occur in sequence from birth to old age. He suggested that each must be successfully mastered before moving on to the next. When a stage is disrupted or unresolved, the failure affects subsequent development.

While the scientific validity of any specific developmental theory is yet to be established, it's clear that the brain develops pathways until a person reaches his early twenties, and that new brain cells can grow throughout life, even into old age. It is also well established that there are certain vulnerable periods of brain development; if an injury or significant stressor occurs during this period, brain development is altered, perhaps permanently. For example, if an injury occurs to the area of the brain that controls language before age six or seven, other areas of the brain can take over so that language function develops normally. An injury that occurs after this period, however, results in permanent language difficulty.

The relevance of this to anxiety disorders can be seen by a patient such as Gail, who lost her mother at two years of age and was raised by a stern, unsympathetic aunt, who made her spend the next year in bed because of an illness that was believed, falsely, to be polio.

At an age when children are learning mastery over themselves and their impulses, Gail not only lost her trusted maternal figure, but was also punished and held back whenever she tried to express her emotions or even get out of bed. It seems quite likely that exposure to this unloving, poorly nurturing environment contributed to the development of obsessive-compulsive behaviors in Gail that worsened as she grew older.

The particular stage when traumas occur in the course of development is believed to produce lifelong effects. In the case of two siblings, a four-year-old girl and her nineteen-year-old brother, who both endured their parents' nasty divorce, the younger child is more likely to develop long-term negative effects. The nineteen-year-old has had more experiences, both good and bad, to draw upon, and his brain is far more developed. The four-year-old, on the other hand, is at a more delicate and susceptible stage of development, when disruption of her safe family circle is far more critical and potentially damaging.

However, just as genetics does not exert total control on whether a person develops an anxiety disorder, neither does early life experience. Indeed, we have all met individuals who have prevailed over the most dire circumstances.

I remember hearing a speech by an elderly African-American minister who chronicled his climb out of childhood abandonment, years of crippling poverty, and drug addiction to a now thriving career helping others.

What accounts for the ability of such people to rise up and overcome so many early obstacles when others are defeated by them?

The minister credited his faith in God and certain life experiences along the way that had given him the boost he needed—particularly people who had believed in him at crucial moments.

He may have also possessed certain temperamental strengths that allowed him to eventually prevail, to turn onto a new path and avoid the potentially permanent effects of exposure to such adverse experiences.

But what *actually* made the difference is part of the mystery—and beauty—of human development.

In fact, whether biology or environment makes us who we are is one of the oldest arguments; recent research has shown us that both are not only important but inextricably linked. In the future, I believe we'll be able to identify people who have a vulnerability for developing anxiety disorders and depression as well as teach them ways of lessening the likelihood that they will ever experience disabling symptoms. Until then, research has taught us that these disorders are neither insurmountable problems nor a failure of individual will. Even if we learn nothing else, these are extremely important lessons.

# 3

# A Partnership of Compassion: Your Role as the Child of an Anxious Parent

A century ago, if your great-grandmother suffered from depression, phobias, posttraumatic stress, or any other anxiety disorder, she might have been labeled weak, crazy, or even possessed by evil spirits.

She might have been kept in a back room, placed in an institution, or treated with such draconian measures as shock treatment or lobotomy. And she most certainly would have been written off, her final years spent in isolation and shame.

Despite sophisticated treatments and vastly improved education, misconceptions about anxiety disorders and depression still persist. If you have an anxious older parent, these old stigmas probably still lurk somewhere—if not in her, then in you or other family members or friends. Helping anxious parents realize that they should not feel shame over these disorders is one of the most important roles you can play.

You also play a vital role in identifying the symptoms that signal the existence of various disorders, as well as in convincing a parent that evaluation and treatment are worth pursuing. Your being informed, supportive, and persistent will greatly increase the likelihood that your anxious parent will ultimately accept the help he needs.

## HOW TO HELP?

In my twenty-five years of practice as a psychiatrist specializing in the maladies of old age, I have encountered many worried children of anxious parents who don't know where to turn for help.

The variations are endless—and distressingly common. A father dies and a mother drifts into clinical depression; a father falls and develops panic attacks that keep him isolated and cut off from the outside world. A mother becomes lost in the vague preoccupations and physical worries that constitute generalized anxiety disorder.

The paradox of being lucky enough to have parents who survive into old age is that you're also more likely to witness their decline. The last thing any of us wants to face is the vulnerability of our parents, heralding as it does the time when we will be without them—as well as echoing our own inevitable aging. We may want to turn away from the melancholy image of a father deteriorating alone in the family house, or a mother who hyperventilates in a doctor's office from a panic attack. It can be tough to watch parents who have comforted us, taught us, and sat securely in the driver's seat throughout our childhoods become frail and vulnerable.

As one daughter put it:

"When my son was young, my heart broke watching all the stumbles and hurts I knew I couldn't control for him, hoping he was well nurtured for all that lays ahead. With my anxious father, I'm learning lessons of a different sort, but they are not unrelated. Half the time, I want to drop everything and just *protect* him. . . ."

But it's not necessary to become a parent's parent in order to help him deal with an anxiety disorder. Rather, it's more beneficial to think of yourself as an advocate and partner in making sure he receives the proper diagnosis and care.

## The Mirror Effect

In the midst of our busy lives, we don't always appreciate the degree of stressful change that older parents routinely face. Spouses die; friends grow ill or move away. Lifelong homes are sold, severing the comfort of old neighborhoods and routines. The independence and status of meaningful work often vanishes. And to top it off, aging bodies become more susceptible to physical illness and the ravages of chronic conditions such as arthritis. All or any of these can produce an accumulative stress load that may trigger anxiety disorders.

Given this, what's remarkable is how *well* most older people cope. Despite the stereotype of late life as a time of psychological weakness, helplessness, and chronic angst, research shows that, as a group, the elderly are *not* overwhelmed with overworry. In fact, studies indicate that older individuals have the highest scores on a sense of life coherence, while middle-aged people report the *highest* worry levels.[1]

Many late-life anxieties mirror those in midlife, and create even more of a challenge for children who face similar issues. Middle age is often a time of job insecurities, bodily changes, and the absence of children in the house—transitions as unsettling as those that occur in late life.

If you're feeling frayed and overextended with career pressures and an awakening sense of mortality, you may be reluctant to stare into the face of your parent's anxieties, mirroring as they do so many of your own.

Mary, an intensive care nurse, told me, "My mother is now right in the middle of everything I fear. She's physically vulnerable, she's worried about money; she's alone since Dad died; she's confused. Sometimes looking at her is like looking at myself, and it's terrifying. There are times when I just don't feel like dealing with her neediness and anxiety. I want to say, 'I'm worried, too! Pull yourself together.' But she's eighty and I'm fifty-seven. She can't do it anymore. And I can."

A stockbroker son told me, "I lost my job and got divorced around the same time my dad slipped into depression. I was in such bad shape myself that I hardly noticed his deteriorating condition . . . it took my sister to make me see that we were *both* depressed. It was a shock to realize that we were struggling with similar issues."

Being aware of these parallels can help you empathize with, and be compassionate toward, an anxious parent.

## A Partnership of Support

It's essential to remember that you can't cure a parent's anxiety disorder any more than he or she can fight it alone. A mother can't be reassured out of her panic attacks or a father reasoned from his obsessive-compulsive symptoms. In the end, a parent needs professional help and guidance, and you may need it, too.

Support and advocacy groups may be as helpful to you as they are to your parent. Accepting this may be as difficult for you as for your mother or father.

Catherine, whose phobic mother lives with her in Maryland, told me, "I found myself saying to my mother, 'You've got to admit you need help,' when I wasn't willing to accept any. I was wearing myself out carrying the burden of my mother's condition all on my shoulders. I finally talked to a counselor and learned to delegate more. I told my brothers: 'This is your mother, too . . . you've got to chip in.' And I decided that if they won't take up the slack, I'll pay for help."

This is not to suggest that reassurance and sympathy aren't vitally important when you are dealing with a parent's anxiety—they are. Listening empathically, being open to hearing about a parent's symptoms and fears—even if it makes you uncomfortable or you think you've heard it before—won't cure a disorder, but it can be therapeutic and comforting. Reassuring a parent that anxiety symptoms are nothing to be ashamed of and that treatment will be a joint effort can all be a great help.

## You *Can* Make a Difference

Having a supportive family can make a tremendous difference in the life of an anxious older parent.

One of my patients, Wilma, is a seventy-seven-year-old woman who'd suffered from panic disorder for years, cycling through different specialists and enduring extensive, overlapping testing. She was able to keep much of this secret from her family, until a call from an emergency room doctor finally alerted her out-of-town daughter to how deeply troubled her mother was. The intervention of her daughter at this point made all the difference in her diagnosis and eventual successful treatment.

Wilma told me: "All the doctors I'd been to throughout the years were unable to find a cause for my spells of rapid heartbeat, difficulty breathing, and nervousness. Most of them basically patted me on the head and told me I was a little old hypochondriac.

"But I *knew* something was wrong with me. I used to be active in church and go on senior trips, but my attacks got so bad that I didn't even want to see my friends anymore. And I didn't want to worry my family until I had something definite to tell them."

She credits her daughter as the main impetus for her eventual treatment and recovery.

"Once my daughter found out what was happening, she wouldn't give up on me. She wouldn't accept that it was all in my head, like some of the doctors said. She drove me to appointments; she sat in, took notes, and asked questions; she urged me to try another medicine when the first one didn't work. I'm glad I finally accepted her help."

# HOW YOU CAN HELP

Understanding what you can and can't do is important during this stage in your life—and your parent's.

Here are some tips to help you navigate:

**Be aware**

Keep track of your elderly parent's moods through phone calls and visits. You may be able to perceive personality or mood changes better than anyone.

If you live far away, ask another family member or trusted friend to report to you regularly. In a facility, establish a relationship with a nurse or staff member who can let you know of a parent's weekly mood and condition. These kinds of alliances are not only essential for information but can also ease the burden on you.

**Assist in recognizing a problem**

Depressed or anxious parents may not even realize that they're suffering from a treatable disorder. They may keep their symptoms to themselves because they're ashamed or don't want to worry you or the rest of the family. Encourage your parent to talk openly about how he's feeling. Once you've established that something may be amiss, be firm in suggesting professional treatment. This is important, since many anxious and depressed elderly never seek or receive help because they feel nothing can be done.

---

**WITH A PARENT RESISTANT TO GOING TO THE DOCTOR:**

- Be patient. Realize you might have to bring up the suggestion several times.
- Make a deal. Try saying, "Let's give it another month; if you don't feel better by then, we'll make an appointment."
- Ask them to see the doctor for you. "I'd feel a lot better if I knew what was going on. Do it for me."

**WITH A PARENT RESISTANT TO PSYCHIATRIC INTERVENTION:**

- Request that a primary-care doctor make a referral.
- Try using words other than "therapist." Suggest instead: "Let's visit a worry specialist."

### Gather information

Once an anxious parent accepts that he needs help, he's often too over-whelmed by symptoms to know where to turn. You may need to be the one to research symptoms, disorders, and treatment options. Educate yourself by reading books, searching the Web, finding local sources of help, and talking to friends or acquaintances in your same situation.

### Arrange exams and assessments

Don't try to diagnose your parent. Do arrange a thorough medical and psychological exam. Have a primary-care physician check out physical symptoms. Explore anxiety symptoms with a geriatric medicine or psychiatry specialist, psychotherapist, social worker, or counselor. Recognize that physical symptoms and anxiety symptoms can be confused. For example, weight loss and fatigue may signal a medical problem, depression, or even a combination of the two. Dementia, drug interactions, and side effects can also complicate diagnosis.

### Accompany a parent to clinician visits

Since an older parent may not be accurate in conveying his medical history, symptoms, or current medication, accompanying him, at least on initial doctor's visits, can be extremely beneficial.

It is important to establish a relationship with your parent's primary-care doctor, who can also be a trusted link if a mental health referral is needed. Let all your parent's clinicians know of your involvement and make sure you are on the list to be called in an emergency.

### Monitor medication

Keep track of what medications your parent is taking, especially when more than one doctor is involved. It's also a good idea to educate yourself about the side effects of your parent's prescription drugs.

### Be persistent

The first or second doctor or treatment you try might not work. You need to be realistic, but keep in mind that most people with anxiety and depression can be helped, no matter what their age. If a parent's symptoms don't improve, ask for a second opinion.

### Share

Your role with an anxious parent should primarily be one of support and advocacy. It's important to understand and respect the wishes of a parent so that you foster autonomy and make joint decisions as much as possible. For example, if a parent is adamantly against either medication or therapy, this should be taken into account when the initial treatment plan is devised.

### Listen

Sometimes what a parent needs most is to be listened to, understood, and soothed. Anxiety symptoms can be terrifying; helping a parent realize that they are the result of syndromes that are treatable and not life-threatening can be a major accomplishment. Simple listening can be one of the most therapeutic activities you can provide.

### Put yourself in your parent's shoes

Try to see your parent from a broader perspective, not as your needy mother or father, but as an older adult struggling with issues of independence and control.

### Reach out

Being the only one involved with your parent's anxiety issues is a sure-fire way of becoming overwhelmed yourself. Since family relationships can become stressed if all the burden of your parent's disorder falls only on your shoulders, you should work to establish relationships with other members of your parent's support network, such as family, friends, clergy, and social workers. Ask for help and support from them and delegate whenever possible. Clearly spell out what needs to be done and what you're already doing. Even though all family members may not share equally, try to make everyone part of the decision-making process.

### Get help

Familiarize yourself with local organizations that offer services for the aging, such as outreach and visitor programs. Locate in-home help, such as a home aide or housekeeper, and make sure that they communicate with you; or investigate senior day-support programs. Hire a geriatric counselor or care manager to handle local arrangements if you're out of town. Have them assist with food shopping, meal and medication delivery, and transportation to appointments.

### Enjoy

Incorporate activities you enjoy into your time with your anxious parent, so that your relationship does not become all dire duty. Make sure you take off time to have dinner, go to a movie, take a walk, or simply talk with your parent. It's important for you to find ways to balance your responsibilities with pleasure.

### Look out for yourself

There's no doubt about it: dealing with a parent's anxiety can make *you* anxious.

Accept what you're able to do and let go of what you can't; becoming so overwhelmed and upset that your own mental health suffers does neither you nor your parent any good.

Find a support group that includes others who are in your same situation. This can provide you with information and advice and give you an outlet for negative feelings. If you're angry, anxious, or impatient, you can transfer these emotions to an already suffering parent, and even exacerbate their problems.

### Reduce your own stress

Set limits when you're feeling overburdened by your parent's problems. Learn to destress through relaxation techniques, yoga, or keeping a journal of your feelings. Taking care of your own needs includes getting adequate rest, exercise, and nutrition, and time away from stressors. Maintain your own social support system. Don't become so involved in your parent's problems that you lose your own identity.

### Let go of guilt

Common feelings that can occur when dealing with an elderly parent's disorder range from impatience, guilt, and exhaustion to the feeling that you can never do enough. Don't take a parent's anxiety or depression personally. Don't fall into the trap of feeling that only you can fix the problem. Also don't grow discouraged if a parent is resistant to your advice. Give yourself credit for what you're able to do, but accept that you can't control a parent's life or future. It's important to remember that an anxiety disorder is no one's fault.

## COMMON MISTAKES CHILDREN MAKE IN DEALING WITH A PARENT'S LATE-LIFE ANXIETY

### Ignoring it

"I had no idea Mom was agoraphobic. She's always been shy!" It's not unusual for adult children to overlook anxiety symptoms because they're so overwhelmed with their own lives; live far away and can't detect symptoms over the phone; don't want to face a parent's vulnerabilities; have a strained relationship with their parent; or are uninformed about the symptoms of anxiety disorders.

### Overreacting

"She forgot my phone number again. She must be getting Alzheimer's!" The opposite of ignoring, overreacting can signal your own fear and cause even more anxiety in a parent. Such a response can also prevent a parent from confiding future symptoms to you—or a doctor.

### Being unsympathetic or angry

"Oh, you'll get over it! You've had nervous spells all your life." If you recognize and receive help for your own frustrations, you're less likely to express anger or lack of sympathy to your parent. Becoming overtly hostile or unsympathetic also signals the erroneous attitude that anxiety is not only a minor matter, but that you are uninterested in dealing with a parent's symptoms.

### Writing them off

"What do you expect, you're eighty-two. Everyone gets nervous when they're old!" Anxiety disorders are not an inevitable part of aging, and they can be treated as successfully in late life as at any other stage. Incorrectly attributing problems to aging can discourage a parent from reporting symptoms and can even contribute to depression.

### Focusing on the physical when the problem is psychological

Elderly parents, especially men, may be more likely to emphasize physical symptoms ("I'm tired all the time; I can't sleep") rather than discussing psychological symptoms ("I'm sad"). This may be because older people experience more physical problems or are unaccustomed to looking at symptoms through a psychological lens. Forcing someone to "admit" that a problem might be psychological makes no sense, but sometimes it can help to personalize a problem. For example, saying, "You know, when I get worried I have the same kind of problem," can help a parent view a symptom differently.

### Not recognizing depression in someone who has become anxious for the first time

Anxiety and depression often coexist in the elderly. While they may need to be diagnosed and treated separately, they are often a single syndrome or condition.

## WHAT CAN I SAY THAT WILL HELP?

It can be difficult to know what to say to an anxious or depressed parent, especially when what he needs most is support and compassion.

Following are some phrases that acknowledge a parent's feelings while signaling your understanding and support.

I'm sorry you're so sad (or anxious). Is there something I can do to help you feel better?

I have sympathy for what you're feeling.

I can see how anxious (or sad) you are.

I love you, no matter what you say or feel.

There are ways we can help you feel better.

These feelings will eventually pass.

Would you like me to sit here and talk with you?

Do you want me to hug you or hold your hand?

I can't experience what you're going through, but I can offer you my compassion.

I'm here for you.

You can count on me.

You mean so much to me.

I won't abandon you.

# PART
# TWO

# 4

# DEPRESSION

## SIGNS YOUR PARENT
## MAY BE DEPRESSED

- Awakens earlier than usual and can't fall back to sleep
- No longer participates in normally enjoyed activities, such as playing cards or visiting family
- Complains of low energy and listlessness
- Cries frequently
- Exhibits lack of interest in eating
- Feels tired all the time
- Loses weight without trying
- Seems forgetful and easily distracted
- Ignores grooming or hygiene
- Won't admit being sad, but focuses on vague aches and pains
- Expresses thoughts that life isn't worth living
- Is preoccupied with guilt and thoughts of failure

In late life, depression is a vastly underdiagnosed and untreated disorder. According to the National Institute of Mental Health, an estimated 7 million Americans over sixty-five suffer from some type of depressive illness, but only a small percentage of them receive treatment. Experts once believed that there was a sharp distinction between anxiety and depression, but it is now clear that they frequently occur together and often are two faces of the same disorder.

Depressive symptoms should never be accepted as an inevitable result of aging. In contrast to natural experiences of grief or transient states of sadness, clinical depression significantly impacts an older person's functioning.

Whenever I see an otherwise healthy older patient slumped in a wheelchair, withdrawn and listless, I think of David.

A retired schoolteacher in his seventies, David had been a lively force in the senior home where he lived after the death of his wife. One of the few men in the facility, David was charming and garrulous, with a large laugh and vivid eyes. He regularly visited the ailing and lonesome, and always left them with some encouragement. He used a cane because of an arthritic hip, and the sight and sound of him tapping down the corridor to spread his cheer was a part of daily life in the home.

Then, everything changed. One winter, an epidemic of flu passed through the senior home, and David caught it. The flu eventually turned into pneumonia and he was hospitalized, near death, for several weeks. When he returned to the senior center, he was a ghost of his former self; his clothes hung on his body, but worse, his formerly animated face was gaunt and expressionless. He didn't want to eat or visit with anyone.

I had been on vacation during the worst of his illness, and when I came upon him, alone in the lobby one afternoon, I barely recognized him.

"I'm kaput," he said, when I sat down to talk to him. "This is the beginning of the end, Doc. I can feel it."

Nothing I said—that he was only seventy-five, that he was fully recovered from pneumonia and could well have many more good years— penetrated his gloom. His general practitioner agreed that David was physically fine, but clearly something was amiss.

During a consult with his son, I said I suspected depression, but the son echoed his father.

"We don't want to intervene in the natural way of things. We have to accept that his life is winding down."

I would be the last person to suggest prolonging the life of someone who is dying from an untreatable disorder, but I was convinced that David need not suffer in this way and that recovery was very possible.

In many settings, this might have been the end of David's story. This is surely the case for many depressed elderly, who are left to deteriorate while their condition is undiagnosed or ignored. Being depressed weakens the immune system, leads to malnutrition, makes people more vulnerable to illnesses and less likely to participate in their own rehabilitation. A serious episode of undiagnosed depression in late life may indeed herald the end.

It's impossible to calculate how many years of productive life are lost because this malady goes untreated. These thoughts occupied me as I walked the halls of the senior home, which now seemed empty and forlorn, bereft of David. I couldn't get him out of my mind.

The next week I visited David in his darkened apartment, where he was spending much of his time alone. He was lying on his bed, and when I drew back the curtain, he winced. He looked even thinner and more gaunt than the last time I'd seen him.

When I mentioned this, he said: "You're a good guy, Doc, but you should use your skills on someone else. I'm useless to anyone now. It's my time. . . ."

"Still, I'd like to ask you some questions about how you're feeling and what you're thinking," I insisted.

He reluctantly agreed.

Upon questioning, he admitted that he couldn't sleep, was uninterested in eating, and had even lost interest in seeing his grandchildren. His thoughts were uniformly despairing and bleak. Not surprisingly his answers met the criteria for major depression.

"I'd like to ask you for a favor," I said when we finished. "There's a pill that I think might make you feel like your old self."

He didn't respond, and he didn't need to. I could feel his resistance.

"Would you take it, just to prove to yourself—and to me—that there's really no hope?"

I could see he wanted to refuse, but a part of him still sparked under the surface. "So how long would I have to take this pill?" he asked.

"A month, two at the most. By then we'll know if it's helping."

He looked at me, and then past me, out the window. "All right, Doc. I'll do it."

Over the next weeks I charted David's progress. At first, little seemed to change. He continued to take his meals in his room and they were still barely touched.

"How do you feel?" I asked when I saw him.

"The same, except for a stomachache."

"That should pass, but let me know if it doesn't."

When I asked whether he was sleeping, he admitted that he was, and until seven A.M., instead of four or five, which had been his recent habit.

"But that's only because I'm so exhausted," he said. Still, this convinced me that we were on the right track.

A few weeks later, I was filling out a chart when I heard something behind me, a sound I realized I hadn't heard for months.

When I turned and saw David in the distance, tapping his way to the dining room, my eyes smarted.

"Good afternoon, Mrs. Golden," I heard him call out. "You're looking beautiful today."

It took nearly four months for David to gain back most of the weight he'd lost and return to his former self. He lived another productive five years, before dying of a sudden heart attack.

If there is a moral to this story, it's not that medicine works for everyone; it's that there are too many elderly who give up too early—and who are given up on by others—because depression has fooled them into believing there is no hope.

David's case shows the many ways depression can be unique in late life.

# HOW DEPRESSION DIFFERS IN SENIORS

## MANY PEOPLE EQUATE BEING OLD WITH BEING SAD

Families often think that if Mom's eighty, has heart disease, and is stuck in a wheelchair, she should be depressed—who wouldn't be?

But this is a dangerous fallacy. Depression is *not* an inevitable side effect of either aging or illness. In fact, the majority of severely ill individuals have no evidence of depression. Yet many families—and doctors—expect the elderly to feel sad, especially if they're medically ill, and don't realize that depression is a treatable disorder.

## DEPRESSION IS MORE LETHAL IN LATE LIFE

Depression tends to be longer-lasting in the elderly. It makes physical illness more serious, and decreases the chances of recovery. By weakening the immune system, it also makes a person more susceptible to new infection.

Depressed elderly are disproportionately likely to kill themselves. Comprising only 13 percent of the population in the United States, people sixty-five and older accounted for 18 percent of all deaths by suicide in 2000, according to the NIMH. The suicide rate for males over sixty-five is the highest in the country. Because they are likely to use lethal methods such as guns, older white males are more likely to succeed than people that use other methods.

## LACK OF TYPICAL SYMPTOMS

One of the most surprising features of late-life depression is that a parent may be as likely to say, "My bones ache, I'm tired all the time" as, "I'm unhappy." In the research I've done on depression we have found that older people with depression are less likely to say that they are sad than younger depressives.[1]

As a result, they may not present to doctors the emotional symptoms that are traditional signs of depression; rather, they complain of lethargy, aches and pains, and an inability to swallow or eat food. Since many doctors aren't trained to take into account bodily symptoms when diagnosing, depression is often overlooked.

Furthermore, depression symptoms such as changes in sleep or diminished energy may be misconstrued as normal manifestations of the aging process or as the result of a physical illness.

## Seniors are less likely to mention depression to doctors

Older people often don't want to "bother" doctors by bringing up depression, or feel that there's a stigma attached to emotional problems. Older men, taught to be strong and unemotional, have a particular problem admitting to depression. In a culture that equates maleness with being rugged and self-sufficient, it can be difficult for an older man to admit he needs help.

## Late-life depression is often precipitated by or coexists with chronic illnesses

Depression often coexists with heart disease, cancer, Alzheimer's, Parkinson's disease, and stroke.

Since these medical problems are more common in late life, families—and doctors—often assume that depression is a normal consequence of these illnesses and leave it untreated.

## Anxiety is sometimes the most prominent symptom of depression in seniors

While depression is not an anxiety disorder, it is common for older parents to suffer from both anxiety and depression at the same time. Occasionally, once the anxiety disorder is treated, the depression also abates. In other cases, the depression remains an issue that must be tackled separately.

# WHAT'S "DEPRESSED"?

Because older parents are so frequently confronted by upsetting change—from the loss of loved ones to moving to a new environment or dealing with a chronic illness—it might seem that it would be difficult to tell when a transitory sadness ends and a clinical depression begins. The distinction, however, is usually quite clear.

Most loss and trauma is followed by a period of sorrow and bereavement. Sad mood is a normal aspect of grief, but mood is usually variable. It's common, for example, for a person to feel suddenly sad when they think of a deceased loved one or see something that is a reminder of him.

Clinical depression, on the other hand, involves a persistent feeling of sadness that either doesn't vary or follows a pattern in which one time of the day, usually the morning, is always worse. The bleak outlook of clinical depression doesn't improve, even when a happy event occurs. A sunny morning, a visit from a grandchild, or a bouquet of flowers won't touch it. It's the persistent nature of depression that differentiates it from situational sadness.

Depression affects the *entire* person. It's as if a gray blanket has been thrown over a patient and cannot be shaken off.

## SOME SYMPTOMS OF DEPRESSION

### Sadness or depressed mood most days

Two-thirds of depressives report being sad or blue, leaving a third who deny this symptom. People who do not report feeling sad often say they are "sick"; that they feel physically ill or "different" in a way that is hard for them to describe.

### Lack of self-confidence, feelings of worthlessness, self-blame, guilt, hopelessness/helplessness

Making statements such as "I'm no good. I'm a burden." Depressed individuals blame themselves for past events, some of which are imagined and some of which are real.

### Persistent physical symptoms

Such as, nearly every day:

- Pain, dizziness, weakness, difficulty swallowing
- Sleep difficulties (oversleeping or insomnia)
- Trouble concentrating
- Agitation or irritability
- Lack of interest or pleasure in usually enjoyed activities
- Loss of energy or fatigue
- Weight loss caused by poor appetite
- Recurring thoughts of death or suicide

# BEING DEPRESSED WITHOUT BEING SAD

So how do you recognize depression in an elderly parent who may be unlikely to complain of a sad or depressed mood?

One red flag is the chronic presence of unexplained physical symptoms such as low energy, poor concentration, early-morning awakening, and poor appetite.

Another is a reduction of self-confidence and the development of self-blame and deprecation.

Mrs. Green was a mild-mannered, soft-spoken, eighty-five-year-old housewife who suffered a serious stroke that left her weak on her right side and unable to speak clearly. Her family was horrified to discover that she had attempted to end her life in the facility where she'd spent two months slowly recuperating. A nurse found her soon after she'd swallowed a cache of pills that she had been hoarding, just in time to have her stomach pumped.

Her children were dumbfounded that their mother could have even considered ending her life.

"I can't believe she'd do such a thing!" her son told me. "She never even told us she was depressed."

But upon further exploration, it turned out that Mrs. Green had been exhibiting certain symptoms of depression that are classic in late life, as well as red flags for suicide.

She was apathetic and listless. She was resistant to physical therapy to re-gain the use of her right side.

"What's the use," she told the therapist. "I'll never be myself again."

According to Mrs. Green's son, this demonstrated a reversal of her nor-mal personality.

When I met with Mrs. Green and asked how she felt, she said, "I don't even know why I'm living anymore. Why don't I die?"

Further questioning revealed that she had a number of other common late-life depressive symptoms, including insomnia, poor appetite, and irri-tability.

Her children were all nearby, showering her with encouragement and support. A daughter had even left her job so that she could devote herself to her mother, bringing in self-help books and tapes and urging her mother to compare herself with others in the rehab facility, who were in far worse shape than she was.

But none of it helped. That's because you can't *talk* someone out of de-pression; they're unable to "snap out of it" by trying harder or as the result of some pithy or compassionate statement on your part. What you *can* do is help them find professional help.

Mrs. Green had no idea that depression was her problem or that anything could be done about it. The despair and inertia of this disorder caused her to believe that her only option was a surrender to suicide. The distorted, bleak outlook of this disorder limited her options and made her think in a self-destructive way.

This shows why it's so important to take seriously any expression of depression or suicidal thought by a parent and to contact a medical professional for help.


## RESISTING THE WORD

Seniors—especially senior men—can be extremely resistant to admitting they are depressed. They may see it as a weakness, a character flaw . . . even sinful, and actively rebel against the label.

This was the case with Jerry, a devout Catholic, who after the death of his wife exhibited a sharp decline in mood and function. His daughter found his home in shambles whenever she visited and her father uncommunicative and morose. But Jerry insisted there was no problem. He wouldn't even allow anyone to use the word "depressed."

"How can I be depressed?" he asked when he met with me. "I'm healthy; I've got a roof over my head. When I was a kid we didn't know from one day to the next what we were going to eat or whether my dad was going to work. Now that's a reason for depression!"

This line of thought is not uncommon in senior parents. But in fact, Jerry *was* depressed, whether he recognized it or not.

I told him, "You wouldn't have talked about your wife's diabetes this way. You accepted that she had an illness and needed help."

But some seniors like Jerry have difficulty accepting that depression *is* an illness, not a character flaw.

His case illustrates what a blinder depression can be—how it limits a person's options.

During our talks, Jerry posed a question I'm often asked: "Why do so many people say they're depressed now? When I grew up, people didn't go around taking pills to make them happy."

Depression has always been a human affliction; descriptions of melancholia can be found in the Bible and Hippocratic writings. It's not that there are more depressed people now, it's that the problem, especially among seniors, had been so vastly unrecognized and undertreated.

In older people, most mental problems were once considered "senility"; this mistake deprived people of care and doomed them to hopelessness. Effective depression medications have been available only for the last fifty years, and newer drugs have made it easier and safer to treat. In the past, all that could be offered were sedatives—or primitive treatments that harmed rather than helped.

In Jerry's case, I made a deal with him; I asked him to try cognitive-behavior therapy for the next several months, along with an antidepressant, as an experiment to see if it made any difference. He took the bait, and when I saw him again two months later, he displayed something I'd never seen before—a smile.

## WHAT CAUSES DEPRESSION?

There are significant elements in life and biology that can trigger depression.

**Specific illnesses** such as heart disease, pancreatic and lung cancer, stroke, Parkinson disease, and Alzheimer's can induce late-life depression. In the cases of both David and Mrs. Green, their physical illnesses probably precipitated the onset of their disorders. It's intriguing that depressions induced by physical illness improve at the same rate as other depressions and positively affect the prognosis of serious illnesses as well.

**Poor eating habits and vitamin deficiencies** can contribute to depression in the elderly. Deficiencies in the B vitamins, especially B-12, are implicated in the genesis of mood disorders. Alcohol and other sedatives, such as barbiturates, Valium, and Restoril, are central nervous system depressants that can induce or worsen symptoms. Marked fluctuations in blood sugar can also produce mood swings and confusion. Omega-3 fatty acids, plentiful in salmon and flax seeds, have been advocated by some experts for boosting mood.

**Chronic pain,** whether from arthritis, back pain, or injury, can induce depression. The mechanism is not known, but it's likely due to persistent stimulation of peripheral nerves causing changes in the brain systems that control pain and pleasure. Some antidepressant medications can diminish chronic pain, even if the person is *not* depressed.

**Social isolation and loneliness.** Depression seems to occur more frequently among those who have few close social ties or emotional relationships. This is true at all ages, but because the death of a spouse is more common in later life, many older parents are alone for the first time in many years and at higher risk for isolation and loneliness.

**Genetics.** Twin, adoption, and family studies carried out in many countries suggest that genetics is a component in the development of depressive disorders.

In a landmark study, researchers at the University of Pittsburgh completed the first survey of the entire human genome and located a number of chromosomal regions they claim hold the genetic keys to a variety of mental illnesses, including major depression and certain addictions. General regions of chromosomes associated with depression in families were discovered, but specific genes remained elusive.[2]

Other research from the University of North Carolina at Chapel Hill suggests that some people with depression have a persistent, biologically based abnormality in their brain's serotonin system, even when the patients are in remission.[3]

Recently, a "short arm" on the gene for the serotonin-transporter protein, a part of the nerve cell that moves serotonin across the nerve-cell membrane, has been linked to an increased risk of developing depression when found with a stressor. Studies are under way to determine whether this is also linked to anxiety. A Johns Hopkins colleague, Dean MacKinnon, has found another genetic linkage in family members who have both panic episodes *and* depression.

Studies like these will be helpful for scientists in developing more effective antidepressant drugs.

**Trauma or stress.** A traumatic event can trigger the initial onset of depression in some individuals. One theory is that stressful events cause enduring changes in brain biology. In the elderly, such an event may be a change in living situation, death of a loved one, development of a serious physical illness, or loss of independence and control.

**Medications.** Drugs such as prednisone and other steroids, reserpine, alphamethyldopa, and benzodiazepines (Valium, Xanax, Ativan) can induce depression.


# TREATMENT

## PSYCHOTHERAPEUTIC TECHNIQUES

Psychotherapeutic methods are a good choice for older parents who are unwilling to take drugs, or for whom medicine doesn't work or causes side effects or drug reactions.

### Best Bets

There is good evidence that older people with depression respond well to **cognitive-behavior therapy,** which trains them to identify and alter negative thoughts and beliefs that lead to depression.

Depressed people are often locked into negative thought patterns. They commonly use all-or-none statements, such as "Nothing in my life is ever good" or "No one ever understands me."

Or as Rita, one of my patients, said, "Nothing I do ever succeeds. I'm useless."

Cognitive therapy demonstrates to someone like Rita that she has the power to change her thinking, and thus her beliefs about herself. Instead of flooding herself with powerful, negative thoughts that keep her locked in a cycle of depression, a therapist would have her first examine the validity of these negative thoughts, then replace them with cognitive coping statements.

To the statement "Nothing I do ever succeeds," a therapist would counter that Rita had a successful, well-paid career and a healthy, long-term marriage.

Whenever the thought "I'm useless" arises in her mind, she would be taught to replace this negative thought with a positive one, such as "I'm a healthy survivor who's coped with many kinds of life situations in my seventy years." She might also be taught to practice thought-stopping, by snapping a rubber band on her wrist whenever negative thoughts occur.

The behavioral component often exposes individuals to situations or objects that they fear or avoid. For example, once Rita began to be gradually exposed to the social groups, volunteering, and activities she had been avoiding, she saw for herself how functional and well liked she was. This boosted her self-esteem and reduced her feelings of depression. She essentially was able to learn from her own successes and to continue to reinforce them by branching out further.

If a parent like Rita is made to see that she has the power to change her thinking—and behavior—depression is more likely to lift.

In fact, cognitive therapy has been shown to impart more lasting benefits in older patients with severe depression than those who take short-term medication alone.

## OTHER NONDRUG THERAPIES

**Psychotherapy** is another option for elderly parents, especially those with mild depression. The primary active ingredient of psychotherapy is discussion with a counselor or other professional who provides encouragement, support, empathic listening, reassurance, and guidance.

Psychotherapy teaches parents to identify mood triggers and to cope with issues that impact their depression. While it may focus on conflicts from childhood that have never been resolved, or on identifying lifelong personality traits that lead to negative interactions, most therapists emphasize the importance of current stressors.

Some seniors may find this kind of therapy too "personal" and may be reluctant to divulge information about private family issues. But a good therapist is often able to develop a rapport and help them overcome this resistance.

**Group therapy** helps sufferers learn how to relate to others and improve relationship problems that might be adding to depression. Its unique benefit is that the participants hear from one another as well as from the therapist. This can be helpful, since conflicts that arise in the group may illustrate problems that members are encountering in real life. Groups are also helpful because of the mutual support they provide—especially when other participants have similar problems or are of similar age.

While group therapy on its own may take several months to be effective, the results are often long-lasting. In my patient David's case, a combination of group therapy with other senior men and medication helped him break out of his depressive cycle.

## PHARMACOLOGICAL TREATMENTS

### Best Bets

I rely on **selective serotonin reuptake inhibitors,** or SSRIs, which "reset" the neurotransmitter system that uses the chemical serotonin, as my first medication choice for treatment of depression as well as anxiety.

These include Celexa, Lexapro, Prozac, Paxil, and Zoloft. For late-life depression, some experts give the highest ratings to Zoloft and Celexa, because they cause fewer interactions with other drugs and fewer withdrawal symptoms, but the evidence for this hypothesis in real life is not yet strong.

Other options I might try are Effexor, a newer drug that impacts both serotonin and norepinephrine, as well as Wellbutrin, a unicyclic that causes fewer sexual side effects.

If one SSRI is ineffective, or causes side effects, it's common to try another or to switch to Wellbutrin or Effexor. It's important for a parent to realize that while the effects of these drugs may be apparent in two weeks, it can take up to eight weeks for their full benefits to be felt.

The side effects of SSRIs are relatively mild. They include insomnia, restlessness, headache, diarrhea, and sexual problems. These effects are less serious than the side effects of older depression drugs, such as the tricyclics.

These drugs should be tapered off gradually under a physician's supervision.

## Other Choices

Older **tricyclic antidepressants** such as Elavil, Tofranil, and Pamelor have proven to be effective for serious depression and may still be used if SSRIs do not work.

Their disadvantages with the elderly, however, are numerous, including cardiac and hypotensive side effects, sedation, dizziness, and high toxicity in overdose. Because of this, they should only be used if one of the newer drugs has failed, unless chronic pain is present.

In my opinion, Elavil and Tofranil should not be used unless Pamelor has failed, since both cause more serious side effects.

**Monoamine oxidase inhibitors (MAOIs)** such as Nardil and Parnate are effective for resistant, chronic depression and depression with anxiety.

But because of their cardiovascular effects (they can cause both high and low blood pressure) and the need to eat a restricted diet to prevent toxicity (no cheese, chocolate, red wine, beer, cured meat), I use these drugs only when an elderly patient with resistant depression doesn't respond to other medications.

**Herbal remedies,** such as St. John's wort (*Hypericum perforatum*) and SAM-e (S-adenosylmethionine) have been advocated as alternative treatments for mild to moderate depression.

St. John's wort extract is believed to affect the reuptake of serotonin in a fashion similar to the SSRIs, but recent studies have shown that it is not as effective for moderate or severe depression.

SAM-e is reported to increase levels of several brain chemicals, including serotonin and dopamine, but it hasn't yet been studied enough to compare it with existing drugs.

Side effects are mild and include stomach upset. Neither should be taken with other antidepressant medications.

## OTHER TREATMENTS

**Electroshock therapy (ECT)** is used for severe depression that is resistant to other treatments and that includes life-threatening behaviors, such as not eating or persistent suicidal thoughts.

ECT is no longer the medieval treatment of the past. A patient now is given general anesthesia and a muscle relaxant before receiving electrical stimulation to the brain. ECT can cause short-term memory loss. The average person requires six to eight treatments, usually given over several weeks. In those with severe depression resistant to other treatments, it has proven to be effective in a high percentage of cases.

**Regular aerobic exercise** produces endorphins, which can help banish depression, promote a sense of well-being, and increase self-esteem. Several studies have shown improvement in mood after exercise in nondepressed individuals, and recent studies have shown this to be true in depressed older individuals as well.

# PROBLEMS THAT CAN MIMIC
# OR COEXIST WITH DEPRESSION

**Anxiety.** When depression and anxiety coexist, it's not uncommon for a parent to complain about anxiety symptoms such as tension and agitation, while denying being sad. Many experts believe that if these symptoms occur in someone who also has depressive symptoms, such as poor appetite, low energy and self-esteem, and early-morning awakening, then depression is usually the primary cause and should be the main focus of treatment.

**"Pseudo" dementia.** In late life this reversible decline in mental functioning may coexist with depression, clouding thinking and making it even more difficult to deal with the disorder. Once depression has lifted, however, memory often improves.

**Recent loss or bereavement.** Grief, a normal response to the loss of friends and loved ones, does *not* equal depression. Depressed people often develop guilt and self-blame, and feel unrealistically responsible for a loss. The grief-stricken, on the other hand, may wish that they had done something different, but don't persistently blame themselves.

Those with depression often fall asleep early, but also wake up early and can't go back to sleep. Those who are grief-stricken may have trouble falling asleep but usually don't awaken early. However, if feelings of grief or sadness persist for two months or more, a parent should always be evaluated for depression.

**Suicidal ideation.** Rates of suicide are higher for white males over sixty-five than for any other age or demographic group in the United States. In fact, suicide rates double in men between ages sixty-five and eighty-five. In addition, older patients with depression are more likely to commit suicide than their younger counterparts. Therefore, thoughts of suicide should be considered a medical emergency and dealt with immediately.

While it's natural for parents in late life to think about the eventuality of death, this is different from having suicidal thoughts. A parent who says "Life isn't worth living" should be taken seriously and asked point-blank: "Are you having thoughts about taking your own life?" A "yes" answer should lead to assessment by a professional as soon as possible.

**Drug side effects.** In addition to the drugs known to induce depression, depressive symptoms can be a side effect of some medications. They include:

- Anticancer drugs (such as Tamoxifen, Velban)
- Antiulcer medication
- High blood pressure medicine
- Pain medications (such as codeine)
- Alcohol

## Questions to Ask Your Parent
## If You Suspect Depression

- Most days:
  Do you feel sad or unhappy?
  Fatigued, listless, hopeless, or uninterested in life?
  Less confident about yourself than usual?
- Have these symptoms kept you from being involved in your usual activities?
- Do you have chronic physical symptoms (weakness, fatigue, loss of appetite, aches and pains, nervousness) that can't be explained by any illness?
- Have you been having feelings of guilt or worthlessness—that you're a burden, or that you're no longer important?
- Are you having more memory problems than usual?
- Do you feel life isn't worth living?
- Have you been drinking more alcohol than usual or combining it with prescription drugs?
- Have you lost a significant amount of weight without dieting?

## HOW YOU CAN HELP

**Facilitate diagnosis and treatment.** If necessary, make the appointment and accompany your parent to the therapist, doctor, or psychiatrist. The very nature of depression can cause inertia; without your help a parent may remain mired in fear and denial.

**Monitor treatment** until the most serious symptoms abate, or find a trusted friend or family member to do so. Encourage your parent to stick with treatment and report any side effects of medication. If one treatment doesn't work, encourage him to seek an alternative.

**Provide emotional support,** understanding, and affection. Talk to your parent, and listen sympathetically. Don't dismiss or denigrate symptoms. Don't feel that recovery is all on your shoulders.

**Be aware** that a father may have special trouble acknowledging feelings of depression. If you suspect your father is depressed, let him know that it's OK to talk to someone about how he's feeling. Help him overcome the stigma that "guys can't seek help."

**Encourage your parent** to get out and participate in activities that were pleasurable before depression—movies, concerts, family events.

**Never ignore suicidal thoughts or remarks.** Report them immediately to a clinician. Insist a parent see a qualified professional.

**Don't take no for an answer.**

## Mood Assessment Scale

This scale was developed as a basic screening measure for depression in older adults.[4, 5] It does not include the physical symptoms that sometimes complicate making a diagnosis. A score above 6 raises the concern that depression might be present; a score above 9 indicates that depression is likely.

1. Are you basically satisfied with your life?
2. Have you dropped many of your activities and interests?
3. Do you feel that your life is empty?
4. Do you often get bored?
5. Are you hopeful about the future?
6. Are you bothered by thoughts you can't get out of your head?
7. Are you in good spirits most of the time?
8. Are you afraid that something bad is going to happen to you?
9. Do you feel happy most of the time?
10. Do you often feel helpless?
11. Do you often get restless and fidgety?
12. Do you prefer to stay at home rather than to go out and do new things?
13. Do you frequently worry about the future?
14. Do you feel you have more problems with memory than most?
15. Do you think it is wonderful to be alive now?
16. Do you often feel downhearted and blue?
17. Do you feel pretty worthless the way you are now?
18. Do you worry a lot about the past?
19. Do you find life very exciting?
20. Is it hard for you to get started on new projects?
21. Do you feel full of energy?
22. Do you feel that your situation is hopeless?
23. Do you think that most people are better off than you are?
24. Do you frequently get upset over little things?

*(continued)*

25. Do you frequently feel like crying?
26. Do you have trouble concentrating?
27. Do you enjoy getting up in the morning?
28. Do you prefer to avoid social gatherings?
29. Is it easy for you to make decisions?
30. Is your mind as clear as it used to be?

This is the original scoring for the scale: One point for each of the answers listed below:

| | | | | | |
|---|---|---|---|---|---|
| 1. no | 6. yes | 11. yes | 16. yes | 21. no | 26. yes |
| 2. yes | 7. no | 12. yes | 17. yes | 22. yes | 27. no |
| 3. yes | 8. yes | 13. yes | 18. yes | 23. yes | 28. yes |
| 4. yes | 9. no | 14. yes | 19. no | 24. yes | 29. no |
| 5. no | 10. yes | 15. no | 20. yes | 25. yes | 30. no |

Cutoff: normal, 0–9; mild depressives, 10–19; severe depressives, 20–30.

## SYMPTOMS OF DEPRESSION

| PHYSIOLOGICAL | BEHAVIORAL | COGNITIVE |
|---|---|---|
| Listlessness | Changes in eating | Persistent sadness and anxiety |
| Fatigue | Difficulty concentrating | Thoughts of suicide or death |
| Sleep problems | Excessive crying | |
| Recurring aches and pain | Loss of interest in activities | Feelings of hopelessness |

# 5

# GENERALIZED ANXIETY DISORDER

## SIGNS YOUR PARENT MAY HAVE GENERALIZED ANXIETY DISORDER (GAD)

- Chronic worry and anxiety over a wide variety of matters for at least six months
- Complaints of persistent muscle tightness, restlessness, stomach upset, fatigue, trouble falling asleep, irritability, and a vague sense of dread
- Always wondering "What if?"
- Going repeatedly to the doctor with various symptoms, even after a clear bill of health
- Becoming impaired in social functioning as a result of worries
- Fearing a dire disease at every minor ache or pain
- Always anticipating disaster
- Blowing up whenever you check on her

■ Inability to "turn off" worry, even though there's awareness that fears are irrational

■ Experiencing trembling, teeth grinding, and dry mouth

It's not so much that a mother with GAD worries about different things than you do, it's that she never stops. She wakes with worry, and she goes to bed with it. She's burdened with a mind that simply won't shut off.

A mother with GAD doesn't experience the world in a normal way. She may be looking at the same event as you are—an upcoming plane trip, a doctor visit—something you may view with mild apprehension, but she conceptualizes and experiences it as terrifying, even catastrophic.

The hallmark of generalized anxiety disorder is this unremitting, relentless worry that cannot be stopped by reasoning or willpower and is not based on any realistic cause.

This disorder may be misdiagnosed as hypochondria, which is defined by the APA as "the fear or belief of serious illness that persists six months or more, despite physician's reassurance." However, with GAD, the worry and anxiety is accompanied by at least three of the following symptoms: edginess, frequent fatigue, trouble concentrating, irritability, tense muscles, or sleep disturbance.

Other common symptoms include heart palpitations, dizziness, frequent urination, headaches, difficulty swallowing, shakiness, aches and pains, and an easy startle response.

Parents with vague, chronic symptoms that cannot be found to have a medical basis are as challenging for their families as for their doctors. Physicians may find themselves in a quandary, because they are reluctant to send a patient for further medical testing on the one hand, but don't want to ignore the patient's worries on the other. In the end, for both moral and legal reasons, doctors may simply continue with tests that are costly, and feed even more into a patient's overworry.

Chronic, nebulous symptoms were bothering my patient George, a seventy-nine-year-old retired businessman who claimed that he hadn't felt well since he'd sold his import/export company three years before. His daughter reported that he had become chronically preoccupied with his health and made frequent trips to a variety of doctors, insisting on diagnostic tests that always came back negative.

"Whenever I see him, he wants me to check a mole on his back or feel his lymph nodes," she told me. "Every month he's worried about a different part of his body. He sits around all day and stews about this kind of stuff."

Physically active throughout his life, George now reported being fatigued all the time and feeling tense in his muscles.

His daughter, who lived in another state, had grown frustrated with him. "He doesn't even ask about his grandkids anymore. Every time I talk to him now, the whole conversation centers on how rotten he feels. He's canceled every visit we've planned for him. Whatever this is, it's ruining all our lives."

When I met with George, a tall, gray-haired man with a melancholy face, he was initially resistant to talking with me. "My daughter thinks something's wrong with my mind," he complained.

When we went over the results of his recent physical, he seemed to intellectually understand that he was healthy, but he still remained visibly anxious. "I see that the numbers are normal, but I just can't believe it," he said.

In our further conversations, he told me more about himself and provided clues to some possible contributors to his condition.

"I'm the only one out of my old gang who still has all his marbles—my friend Bud has Alzheimer's and doesn't even recognize me when I visit; my other friend Jim is in a nursing home because of a stroke. He can't even talk or feed himself. All the rest—they're gone.

"I used to run my own business—forty people were dependent on me; I got up at six in the morning and went to bed at eleven at night. I had so much to do that I hardly had time to read the paper. Now I don't have any reason to get up. And I can't get to sleep, I'm so keyed up and upset."

George exhibited many of the classic symptoms of GAD: muscle tightness; a persistent, vague sense of dread; and fluctuating physical symptoms.

He admitted that he'd had bouts of anxiety in his younger years, but had been able to keep them in check. He acknowledged that loss of status and a general feeling of purposelessness may have triggered problems that he'd previously been able to handle.

"It may be all in my mind," he told me, "but it *feels* real to me."

Many GAD sufferers realize that their fears are irrational, but that doesn't mean they can turn them off. No matter how hard they try, their cycle of worry cannot be broken by reasoning or willpower. Telling a parent to "snap out of it," as George's daughter tried, is a waste of time. Because of this, GAD is an exhausting disorder for both patient and family and can result in isolation, loneliness, and demoralization.

It's not unusual for sufferers to cycle through a number of doctors and specialists for a variety of physical complaints, from shortness of breath to dizziness, insomnia, and vague aches and pains.

Before George came to see me, he had seen a cardiologist, several neurologists, and a pulmonary specialist and was resentful when doctors were unable to detect anything physically wrong with him. The closest George received to a diagnosis was when a doctor told his daughter, "He's getting old; his systems are failing."

In George's case, it turned out that the doctors were as blind to his condition as everyone else. Late-life GAD is a syndrome that is not always easy to diagnose or differentiate from physical problems or other conditions, such as dementia and depression. This is one of the reasons why it is important to make sure an elderly parent's therapist and doctor are specially trained in geriatrics.

## NORMAL WORRY VERSUS GAD

There are legitimate reasons to experience spells of anxiety and worry in late life, a time when an elderly parent may be regularly confronted with challenges and losses. If a father reacts to the news that he has leukemia with withdrawal and insomnia, or a mother who has just lost a best friend becomes withdrawn and morose, these are understandable responses.

A majority of parents will face such challenges and traumas with grief and some degree of anxiety, but eventually bounce back to return to their normal life.

But with GAD there is none of this adaptability; the elasticity has gone out of their response. There is no beginning or end to their worry—it takes on a life of its own and becomes chronic, persistent, and overwhelming. When one fear is resolved, another one takes its place in an exhausting, unending cycle.

A GAD worrier is often on edge and fretful about a number of matters all at the same time. She can never really relax.

Although GAD is common in late life—up to 7 percent of the elderly population suffer from it,[1] and it's more frequent among women than men—it's only recently that the disorder has been recognized as a bona fide syndrome, rather than a personality trait.

"We always teased my mother about her worrying," a son told me about his mother, Mrs. Baker. "It was a joke in our family, what a worrywart she was. If her plane wasn't going to crash, the wheels were going to fall off her car while she was driving. You name it, she'd worry about it. And this isn't even mentioning her hundreds of imagined illnesses. Other kids grew up with encyclopedias. We grew up with the *Merck Manual.* We knew the symptoms of every disease, and my mother had them all."

Mrs. Baker had spent much of her adult life paralyzed by fear, always imagining the worst possible outcome. She was scared to travel, change jobs, even host a dinner party at her house. Nevertheless, she successfully raised her children, worked as an office manager, and saved for her retirement.

"As she got older, Mom's behavior wasn't so funny anymore," her son continued. "After she moved into a retirement home, it got really bad. She became totally isolated and fearful. One day when I visited, I came upon her sitting by herself with a long face.

"'What's wrong, Ma?' I asked her, and she said, with a perfectly straight face, 'I think I have end-stage liver disease.' And it hit me all at once that this really *was* an illness that needed to be addressed. She'd had this albatross around her neck all these years. I couldn't allow her to be in pain without dealing with it. That's when I finally insisted we find a therapist."

## SICK *AND* ANXIOUS

When GAD coexists with a physical illness, it complicates both diagnosis and treatment. Having an anxiety disorder *along with* a physical ailment can be a double burden for an elderly parent, placing a heavy load on an already stressed body.

Illness often obscures the coexistence of GAD, and makes coping even more challenging. Family members may assume that anxiety is an understandable component of being ill and that there's no need for it to be separately treated. But research shows that most people who are ill are *not* depressed and anxious. GAD is a distinct disorder, separate from whatever other illness a parent is suffering from. And it is just as essential to treat.

Mattie had always been a chronic worrier, but at the age of eighty-one, when she discovered a breast lump, her condition significantly worsened. She wouldn't leave the house or get out of bed, and she didn't tell anyone about her finding for nearly six months. When she finally told her daughter about the breast lump, she refused to see a doctor. "What if they tell me I'm dying? I won't be able to handle it," she later admitted she thought.

After weeks of pressure from her family, Mattie finally agreed to an appointment with a breast specialist, where a mammogram and biopsy confirmed she had an early stage of cancer.

This news confirmed all her long-held anxieties. "What's the use?" she said when radiation and chemotherapy were recommended. "I'm never going to make it anyhow."

Even when her daughter did some research on the Internet and presented her with compelling information that a positive outcome was very possible if she received timely treatment, Mattie remained paralyzed. "I understand what you're saying to me, I just don't believe it's true," she said. This is a common feature of generalized anxiety disorders; even though a patient may intellectually realize that her fears are unreasonable, she is unable to overcome them.

At this point, Mattie's daughter considered her mother's GAD life-threatening; without treatment, her mother's breast cancer would likely spread.

She made an appointment with me to see Mattie, and I put her on Ativan (lorazepam) on the mornings she was due for chemotherapy and radiation. Her rapidly improved mood countered her paralysis and allowed her to begin treatment.

A year later, she had completed radiation and chemo and was found cancer-free. During the year, she had also begun cognitive-behavior therapy, which helped her learn techniques to cope with stress. Armed with these new methods of coping, she was eventually able to get off her medication.

## WHAT CAUSES GAD?

Like most anxiety syndromes, GAD results from a complex confluence of genes, experience, and stress; it's not always easy—or possible—to sort out the exact cause of a patient's disorder. However, there are a number of factors that contribute to the development of GAD.

### AGING CHALLENGES

Older parents are routinely confronted with some of life's most stressful challenges. They frequently have to cope with threats to their independence and sense of control, as well as declines in physical and mental competence. They also regularly face the deaths of close friends and other loved ones. And there are often financial concerns, since many seniors are no longer employed. All or any of these can produce an accumulative stress load that may trigger GAD in those who have a tendency to overworry.

### TRAUMAS

Some experts believe that illnesses, such as strokes, heart attacks, and cancer, may precipitate GAD. Certainly this disorder can be aggravated by serious illnesses and dire medical conditions. But the situational anxiety that is often a component of serious illness does not necessarily herald the development of GAD.

Research suggests that early-childhood traumas may increase the chances of developing GAD. I believe it likely that individuals with a constitutional vulnerability to worry develop GAD if they have experienced a significant trauma early in life.

## GAD AND GENETICS

Since GAD often shows up in several members of a family, it is likely that there is a genetic component to the disorder. Studies of identical twins show that if one twin has an anxiety disorder, the other is much more likely to suffer from one also, even if the twins have been raised separately. This likelihood is much lower in fraternal twins, who have the genetic similarity of siblings, rather than the exact same genetic makeup of identical twins. What seems to be inherited is an overreactive, vulnerable personality type that tends to worry to an extreme degree and for a longer period of time than someone without the vulnerability.[2]

## BIOCHEMISTRY

GAD is believed to occur when there is a malfunction of the brain systems that depend on the neurotransmitter gamma aminobutyric acid (GABA). Abnormalities in the neurotransmitter serotonin have also been implicated. A recent study demonstrated that a gene that makes a protein necessary for moving serotonin across brain cell membranes can affect how an individual responds to stress, and that this is likely how genetics and environment interact.[3]

## DEMENTIA

Dementia, a common disorder in late life, can lead to the development of GAD, as well as panic. Early symptoms of memory loss and other cognitive impairments may cause a parent to become isolated and fearful, yet unaware that his memory is failing.

# TREATMENT

A treatment program should be personalized to suit the unique needs of a parent. Most research suggests that a combination of psychotherapy and pharmacological treatments is more effective in the long run than either on its own.

However, since many elderly already suffer from other medical conditions that require them to take a number of medicines, psychotherapy and other nondrug methods are a good first start.

## PSYCHOTHERAPEUTIC TECHNIQUES

### Best Bets

In general, I like to start a parent suffering from GAD with **cognitive-behavior therapy.**

The basic thrust of CBT is that in order to improve symptoms, you need to change both the person's thinking pattern *and* how he behaves. CBT helps a parent learn to view events from a new perspective and find fresh ways to cope with chronic anxiety and fear.

The theory behind CBT suggests that GAD sufferers react to dangers that they have erroneously perceived as harmful, on the basis of their tendency to view the world—and themselves—in a distorted, negative way. Cognitive-behavioral therapy teaches techniques that focus on changing a parent's negative thinking and coming up with new ways of reframing a problem.

My patient George was taught how to manage his anxiety symptoms by combating his anxiety-producing thoughts. He learned to replace, or reframe, his chronic progression from "I have a headache, it's probably a brain tumor, I better go to the emergency room," with a positive replacement, such as: "I've had headaches before; they've never been the result of a tumor and have always gone away. This is anxiety, and if I relax, the headache will disappear without a trip to the hospital."

Combined with behavior techniques, this helped him combat his chronic overworry.

**Behavioral therapy** helps parents locate and change behaviors that maintain their syndrome. These techniques help them learn to avoid certain situations and environments that trigger stress responses.

Mrs. Baker was paralyzed with worry whenever her son went away on his monthly business trips. She isolated herself in her apartment and monitored the news channels, terrified that his plane would encounter dangerous weather or be attacked by terrorists. In behavioral therapy, she was taught alternative behaviors that aided her at this time of the month. She preplanned pleasurable distractions—visits to friends and other social engagements—that got her out of the house, and she began a regular exercise program. Whenever she wanted to turn on the news channel or phone him overseas, she was instructed to distract herself with another activity—a brisk walk or listening to a book on tape, for example.

In **interpersonal psychotherapy,** GAD patients can work with a therapist to discuss and resolve conflicts and problems that may be haunting their lives. Psychotherapy can provide benefits that many elderly are missing—including support, education, empathic listening, reassurance, guidance, and a means of breaking out of isolation.

Research shows that older individuals are as likely as younger people to change with this kind of therapy. Improving relationships with a spouse or children, for example, can go a long way toward combating the paralyzing worry of GAD. These same approaches and issues can take place in group therapy, which has the added advantage of providing peer support.

However, some older parents may be strongly opposed to this type of therapy, finding it too threatening, intrusive, or "personal."

**Calming therapies** are also effective for alleviating GAD symptoms. Relaxation techniques, including progressive relaxation, biofeedback, abdominal breathing, and meditation all help banish stress by teaching a person steps to take to combat the physical sensations that are a part of anxiety.

A regular exercise regimen is also an excellent way to promote relaxation. My patient George was helped by a combination of CBT methods, including guided visualization techniques, where he transported himself to a calming setting; deep abdominal breathing; and a vigorous workout every other day. These interventions seemed to help him restore a sense of control over his life and his symptoms.

## PHARMACOLOGICAL TREATMENTS

### Best Bets

**Selective serotonin reuptake inhibitors (SSRIs),** commonly referred to as antidepressants, are also effective for a wide range of anxiety disorders, including GAD. SSRIs are believed to work by restoring the balance of the brain chemical serotonin.

In a wide number of studies, these drugs are found to be effective, with less serious side effects (including nausea, constipation, insomnia, sexual dysfunction) than older drugs like Valium, and with fewer withdrawal problems. Because of this, they're my first choice for treating GAD in the elderly. Zoloft, Lexapro, and Paxil are SSRIs specifically approved for GAD, but others seem just as effective.

A newer dual-action drug, Effexor, has also been approved for use in GAD treatment; it boosts both serotonin and norepinephrine and is therefore known as an SSNRI. The extended-release form is convenient because it need be taken only once a day.

Patients should be reminded that they may feel better in as little as two weeks, but that it can take up to eight weeks for the full effects of an SSRI to be felt, especially since the dosage may need to be increased gradually. Depending upon the drug, many side effects abate after the first few weeks of treatment. If one SSRI is not effective, another may be, or an SSNRI might be tried. All these medications should be tapered off slowly, under a doctor's supervision.

**Buspirone (BuSpar)** is a nonaddictive antianxiety drug that is approved for the treatment of GAD. Its benefits with the elderly include the fact that it has few side effects and can be taken by those with medical problems.

BuSpar is usually given in divided doses several times a day. It is not as fast-acting as benzodiazepines (Ativan, Valium, Xanax, and related drugs), and may take two continuous weeks of therapy before an effect is felt. It is safer than benzodiazepines, but in my experience not as effective as SSRIs or SSNRIs.

## Other Choices

**Benzodiazepines** such as Klonopin, Xanax, Valium, and Ativan can be effective for a patient like Mattie, who was paralyzed by her GAD and needed rapid relief in order to begin her cancer treatment. In general, shorter-acting drugs such as Ativan are a better idea for the elderly than longer-acting ones such as Valium or Klonopin. Lower doses are also recommended for older individuals.

These medications should only be used for short-term interventions in the elderly because of their addictive properties and troublesome side effects, including sedation, memory impairment, and unsteadiness. If a benzodiazepine has been used for any extended period, the dosage should be tapered off gradually. Withdrawal reactions can be life-threatening. Symptoms include tremulousness, anxiety, lethargy, delirium, and seizures. Tapering off from benzodiazepines must be done under the supervision of a doctor.

# PROBLEMS THAT CAN MIMIC OR COEXIST WITH GAD

**Medical conditions** such as hyperthyroidism (too much thyroid hormone produced by the body), head trauma, brain infections, heartbeat irregularities, and asthma have been linked to GAD. These disorders can cause a variety of anxiety-like symptoms, from tension to difficulty breathing to a rapidly beating heart.

**Nutrition.** Lack of a balanced diet in late life can alter electrolyte function and blood-sugar levels, producing a wide variety of symptoms that may be read as anxiety, including shakiness, trembling, weakness, and emotional upset. Excessive caffeine and nicotine cause heart palpitations, muscle twitching, and feelings of tension and overstimulation—all symptoms of GAD.

**Alcohol abuse.** People who are chronically anxious often self-medicate with alcohol. Alcohol usage and withdrawal may also produce GAD symptoms. A parent who seems shaky or nervous may be undergoing alcohol withdrawal.

**Medication usage.** Patients who take antianxiety medications such as Valium, Xanax, and Ativan may become addicted. Withdrawal symptoms cause increased anxiety and lead to further increases in doses, ultimately compounding the problem even more. A patient may also have several prescriptions from different doctors, be overmedicating, or combining different medicines; this, too, can heighten the risk of physical addiction.

**Other psychiatric disorders.** GAD is a condition that often coexists with other mood and anxiety disorders. Some experts believe that 50 percent of patients with GAD also have another mental disorder, such as panic disorder, dementia, and especially depression.[4]

## Questions to Ask Your Parent If You Suspect GAD

- Have you been overcome with worry for no real reason?
- Did something particular trigger these worries?
- Do you feel any three of these symptoms at the same time as the increased worry: edginess, frequent fatigue, trouble concentrating, irritability, tense muscles, or sleep disturbance?
- How have these worries changed your everyday habits?
- Are you secretly frightened about having an illness?
- Have you been visiting a number of doctors for varying symptoms?
- Have you altered your medications or the way you've been taking them?
- Have you changed your diet or your caffeine or alcohol consumption?

## HOW YOU CAN HELP

**Make sure your parent receives a medical evaluation** to rule out physical ailments.

**Validate, don't dismiss symptoms and complaints.** Avoid saying things like: "Snap out of it. Don't worry. Everything will be all right." Instead, try: "I know you're scared. Is there anything I can do to help you?"

**Once diagnosed,** remind parents that GAD is an anxiety disorder and that the symptoms aren't life-threatening.

For example, say: "Mom, we know you feel bad, but the good news is that Dr. Cole says you have an anxiety disorder, not lung disease, and with the right treatment you can feel a lot better."

**Divert attention from symptoms** by encouraging a parent to participate in a relaxation or physical exercise with you. Reinforce positive outcomes: "See, don't you feel better since we took our walk?"

**Monitor doctor's visits,** medical reports, and medication to ensure that a parent isn't receiving overlapping medication or duplicate testing.

### SYMPTOMS OF GENERALIZED ANXIETY DISORDER

| PHYSIOLOGICAL | BEHAVIORAL | COGNITIVE |
|---|---|---|
| Palpitations | Frequent doctor's visits | Excessive, uncontrollable worry |
| Restlessness | Shortness of breath | |
| | | Difficulty concentrating |
| Muscle tension | Impaired social and work functioning | |
| Disordered sleep | | |
| | Irritability | |

# 6

# OBSESSIVE-COMPULSIVE DISORDER

## SIGNS YOUR PARENT MAY HAVE OBSESSIVE-COMPULSIVE DISORDER

- Has intrusive thoughts and impulses that cause distress
- Is fixated on "rules" about how things should be
- Can't stop certain mental processes, such as counting backward from one hundred
- Feels terrible pressure to perform ritualized actions, such as checking the oven and locks
- Insists on having things in order or in a certain pattern
- Worries about germs and contamination
- Hoards objects
- Exhibits obsessions/compulsions that take up at least an hour or more a day and interfere with daily functioning
- Realizes that these thoughts and actions aren't rational, but still can't stop them

Obsessive-compulsive disorder is one of the fiercest and most disturbing syndromes to suffer from—or to deal with in a loved one. A parent with

OCD is saddled with intrusive thoughts and impulses that won't go away and that cause him to perform repetitive, ritualistic behaviors even though he realizes that they make no sense.

This is a textbook description, but it's hard to be clinical when your father is stuck in the bathroom, cleansing himself in an elaborate, hour-long ritual that has caused the skin on his hands to chafe and bleed. Or when your mother is stalled in front of her doorway, repeatedly touching a certain spot on the wood before she can go outside. Symptoms like these can make OCD a life ruler, a strong and disturbing disorder.

Before modern treatment, people with OCD were often considered crazy or possessed by demons. In fact, until the nineteenth century, the disorder was often treated by exorcism, and as late as the 1940s, lobotomies were regularly performed.

Once believed to be rare, OCD afflicts as many as one in fifty Americans and is evenly distributed among sex, race, and economic backgrounds.[1]

Since OCD has only recently been recognized as treatable, older parents may be accustomed to having their symptoms ignored or misunderstood. They may also be expert at camouflaging them until they begin to interfere with daily functioning, as happened with Dan's mother, Sylvia.

Eighty-one-year-old Sylvia lived alone in the old family house in rural Ohio, while Dan lived and worked several hours away in Cleveland. On his weekly visits, Dan began noticing the acceleration of several odd behaviors in his mother. First, she took an extensive amount of time getting ready in the morning and had to dress herself in a particular order, bottom to top, left before right, buttons before zippers. If interrupted at any point in her regimen—if the phone rang or Dan asked her a question—she had to begin the process all over again. This meant that it often took her several hours to dress every day.

Dan admitted: "She always had strange tendencies that used to drive my dad crazy, but he dealt with it somehow. But now that he's gone, there's no one for her to hide behind."

Sylvia had also begun to hoard all kinds of objects, filling her house with carefully arranged piles of aluminum foil, junk mail, and newspapers.

Dan said: "Whenever I visited, I could barely walk through the kitchen and dining room for the stacks of newspapers and magazines. Every surface was stacked. There wasn't even any place to sit. When I asked: 'Why are you keeping all this, Mom?' she said: 'I might write a cookbook someday, so I can't throw anything away that has a recipe on it.'"

Eventually it became obvious to Dan that this was a behavior his mother simply couldn't control. When he picked up a pile of papers and headed out to the garbage one afternoon, his mother screamed at him: "Don't do that, Dan! Please, stop!"

"I looked her in the eye and said, 'Mom, you've got to stop this! It's crazy.' And I saw that she understood me but that it didn't matter. It was as if there were some terrible thing trapped in her that was ruling her life."

Dan is in the same boat as many adult children whose parents are suffering from the sometimes bizarre symptoms of OCD. It can be frustrating for family members to figure out how to help. This is further complicated by the fact that elderly parents may hide OCD symptoms because they are ashamed or afraid that these symptoms mean they're demented or crazy. And if they live alone, like Sylvia, they may be able to keep their symptoms secret for longer.

## PERSONALITY VERSUS DISORDER

Everyone possesses some degree of perfectionism. We're all somewhere on a continuum from being rigid and perfectionist to sloppy and lax. While your spouse may not be able to tolerate a single dirty dish in the sink, it may not bother you in the least, while an unmade bed drives you up the wall.

For most of us, these tendencies don't affect our lives adversely. In fact, perfectionist qualities are valued in many situations; you probably don't mind if your child is meticulous with her algebra homework or if a surgeon is especially careful when he's operating on you.

But a parent with obsessive-compulsive disorder is suffering from an illness that is categorically different from normal elements of perfectionism. He is laboring under conditions of a serious disorder that rarely disappears on its own.

Depression is a good parallel model. Everyone becomes discouraged and low at times, but clinical depression isn't simply an extreme bout of sadness. Instead, the mood thermostat becomes stuck in the depressed position no matter what happens. A person could win the lottery and still feel unhappy.

It's the same with obsessive-compulsive disorder. A person can wash for weeks and never feel clean enough to be really satisfied. The condition does not exist on dirty hands but, literally, in the mind.

It's important to differentiate between a tendency toward OCD traits, which are often worsened by stress and may be treated with counseling, and the full-blown disorder, which almost always requires medication.

Sixty-nine-year-old Mark was a former navy officer who had always been a stickler for order and control. During a routine physical, a hard nodule was discovered on his prostate gland. After a biopsy, he was scheduled to return in a week for the results.

As the days progressed, Mark became even more rigid and controlling, yelling at his wife and adult children because they weren't doing things exactly the way he wanted them. His daughter reported, "He wanted everything in the house placed in its designated location—right down to the pots and pans in the kitchen. It was ridiculous, but he got crazy about it. I thought he was going to have a stroke when I moved a dining room chair from its correct spot."

His daughter was able to recognize that the stress of the prostate biopsy was exacerbating a personality trait Mark had always had.

She took him aside and said: "Dad, I know you're really uptight about this procedure, but it's starting to spill over in the way you relate to everyone. Try counting to five before you get so upset at Mom. And why don't you talk to Uncle Jim about what he went through with his prostate biopsy."

This small intervention was enough to curb Mark's anxiety until the biopsy results came in. Luckily, they were negative, and his extreme behaviors disappeared. Had the results been positive, his daughter had already located a counselor for Mark to talk to in order to help him deal with his stress.

Such counseling would target Mark's fears about cancer and the future, and help him realize that when he's under pressure he becomes more rigid and more likely to upset the people he loves.

In this case, treatment might be as simple as recognizing that such behavior was Mark's lifelong pattern, that stress exaggerated it, and that minimizing such stress, along with counseling, could alleviate much of the problem.

This type of approach would not have worked, however, if Mark had a full-blown case of obsessive-compulsive disorder, like seventy-seven-year-old Adam, who insisted that he and each member of his family take a shower whenever they entered his house. Adam's contamination obsession had been something he'd battled all his life. Medication had helped him remain functional until after a heart attack, when he went off his meds and his symptoms returned full force.

"Even if we go outside to get his mail, or move his garbage can to the curb, he insists we need to shower again. We began dreading going over and visiting," his grandson reported. "It sounds humorous, but he became a real nightmare to deal with."

It was only after Adam began taking medication on a regular basis that these behaviors abated and his quality of life improved.

## LIFE'S RITUALS

Worries, ritualistic behaviors, and superstitions are a part of daily life, but it's one thing to avoid walking under a ladder or trying to avoid a crack in the sidewalk, and quite another to spend your days lining up furniture or hoarding laundry lint.

In OCD, the processing of information in the brain has gone amok; it becomes snagged on an urge or thought and can't become free of it. Celeste was a devout Catholic whose life revolved around the rituals of her religion. An important part of her daily routine involved attending mass and saying the rosary. Such repetitive, ritualistic behaviors can be fulfilling and have a beneficial effect on an elderly parent's life. But they aren't the same as a compulsion. If Celeste had to miss services due to a storm, for example, she wouldn't feel an overwhelming pressure to head out into dangerous weather.

She would be able to say to herself: "I'm disappointed that I can't go to mass because of the snow, but there's nothing I can do about it. I'll go to-morrow."

Her behavior is in opposition to that of Hilda, who could not go to the grocery store without traversing it in a particular route—from dairy, through meat, to produce. If she missed any station along her route, she had to begin all over again at the front door. This would not have been such a problem except that her children had to accompany her on these grocery trips, and a single visit often consumed most of the day.

Hilda, unlike Celeste, could not say, "I bypassed the dairy section today; it's okay. I'll go there next time." She felt that she *had to* adhere to this pattern. If asked why, she could only say that her actions had to do with "feeling safe."

Celeste's religious rituals had meaning to her and were a pleasurable part of her life. Hilda's actions, on the other hand, provided short-term relief, but did not give her pleasure. This is a crucial difference between an OCD tendency and a disorder.

## A DISORDER OF DOUBT

OCD is a doubting disorder, where a parent can never feel certain that what he is focused on is taken care of adequately. Often there is intense attention to small, specific things—hours can be spent on grooming rituals, countings, or checkings. The anxiety can increase to terrifying levels if the compulsion is not allowed to take place.

The most common obsessions center on:

**Contamination,** such as saliva, bodily secretions, dust, or germs. Because a parent experiences overwhelming disgust or anxiety when in the presence of these items, he feels compelled to frequently wash himself or remain inside the house where he's "safe."

**Doubting,** where car brakes, locks, and stoves need to be constantly checked. This compulsion is connected with fear and a chronic guilt that something important has been forgotten or overlooked.

**Orderliness or preciseness,** which can result in a parent taking hours to dress, eat, or count or line up objects.

Another common variation is for a parent to be consumed with obsessional worry that doesn't necessarily cause any compulsion but is debilitating on its own. One of my patients, Jim, was obsessed with the notion that he'd done something wrong and would be sent to jail. This caused him great anguish, even though he realized, intellectually, that this made no sense. He said, "I know I'm not doing anything illegal. I pay my taxes; I don't even go through yellow lights. But I still have this worry in my mind that I've done something wrong."

Jim realized his fears were foolish, but that didn't mean he could keep from ruminating and rehashing his daily interactions in a fruitless search for illegalities. These obsessions kept him suffering and isolated, unable to enjoy his life.

## WHAT CAUSES OCD?

### GENETICS

Studies suggest that there is an inherited predisposition in the development of OCD. If one person in a family suffers from the disorder, there is a greater chance that another immediate family member will also have it. In fact, family studies have shown that 35 percent of first-degree relatives of OCD patients also have the disorder.[2]

### TRIGGERING ILLNESS

The onset of OCD can be precipitated by an illness, such as rheumatic fever, which is due to a streptococcal infection. Strep antibodies attack a particular part of the brain, which can result in the development of repetitive behaviors and other OCD symptoms.

Another triggering illness is influenza. After the epidemic of 1918, which killed 20 million people, some people developed encephalitis and manifested OCD-like behaviors upon recovery.

### NEUROBIOLOGY

OCD sufferers are believed not only to have abnormal brain chemistry, but also abnormal activity in specific areas of the brain. OCD has been linked with chemical imbalances that result in communication difficulties between the frontal lobe and deeper regions that regulate repetitive behavior.

EEG studies of OCD sufferers have also shown a higher incidence of brain activity in portions of the brain associated with anxiety, habit forming, and skill learning.[3]

Low levels of the brain chemical serotonin—or a disturbance in serotonin metabolism—have also been implicated in OCD. This has been reinforced by the fact that OCD sufferers often improve when they take SSRIs, which boost serotonin reuptake.[4]

### TRAUMA

OCD may be precipitated by a trauma, such as the death of a loved one or a serious illness. It also appears to be worsened by accumulated stress and psychological factors.

## TREATMENT

Anyone who has tried to "reason" with an OCD patient understands why Freud stated that true obsessive-compulsive disorder was the one problem that psychotherapy couldn't solve. In fact, until the 1940s, full frontal lobotomies were employed to "cure" OCD sufferers.

Medication is a central part of OCD treatment, along with the insight-oriented treatments that constitute cognitive-behavior therapy

## PSYCHOTHERAPEUTIC TECHNIQUES

**Cognitive-behavior therapy** is beneficial in treating obsessions and compulsions, especially in conjunction with medication.

**Behavioral therapy** is focused on bringing a patient into systematic encounters with dread objects or situations. Based on the belief that a gradual exposure to a feared object generally lessens its power, this type of therapy can involve imaginary or literal exposure. By taking small, incremental steps toward a feared object or situation, a patient is able to face and ultimately gain control of his fear.

This therapy is most helpful when coupled with **response prevention,** which is aimed toward compulsions.

In response prevention, a patient is not only exposed to a feared situation or object, such as dirty money, but his compulsive behavior is blocked. In the case of a contamination phobia, a patient might be asked to handle money and then be prohibited from immediately washing his hands. In the case of Sylvia, whose laborious dressing rituals had to be started all over again if she was interrupted, response prevention might involve distracting her a little, then preventing her from starting her regime again; then distracting her more, and preventing her again, and so on.

Adam, a constant showerer, was instructed to reduce his washing rituals from four to three then two times daily over several months. Eventually he was able to shower once a day. He was also discouraged from asking family members to clean themselves when entering his house. When they entered and he felt the urge to ask them to shower, he went to his room and performed progressive relaxation and deep-breathing techniques until the urge passed.

**Cognitive therapy** helps a parent evaluate fears and come up with new methods of handling them. This kind of therapy can assist a parent in reducing the kind of catastrophic thinking that is linked with OCD.

CT includes cognitive restructuring, in which a parent is helped to replace an obsessive thought ("What if I've forgotten to turn off the gas? The house might burn down") with a less exaggerated one ("In forty years, I have always turned off the gas when I vacated the house; I will check it once, then leave)." The repetition of such reassuring statements can be helpful in breaking the OCD loop of frantic, out-of-control checking behaviors.

**Thought-stopping** techniques are also used, such as snapping a rubber band worn around the wrist whenever an unwanted thought enters a patient's mind. This technique helped Adam, for example, whose contamination obsessions were ruling his life. Whenever he had the thought "That's filthy! That's contaminated!" he was instructed to snap the rubber band to stop the thought.

## PHARMACOLOGICAL TREATMENTS

### *Best Bets*

The most long-used and widely studied drug for treating OCD is the SRI **clomipramine.** A nonselective SRI, this drug affects both serotonin and norepinephrine neurotransmitters in the brain. However, since clomipramine has many side effects, including tremors, dizziness, and sedative and cardiac effects that can cause significant problems in older individuals, I only recommend it when other medications have failed.

I prefer using **SSRIs,** which increase the availability of the neurotransmitter serotonin at brain synapses. They have less serious side effects, require one dose a day, and are not addictive.

SSRIs that are approved for OCD include Prozac, Paxil, Zoloft, and Luvox. While SSRIs have their own side effects, including weight gain and insomnia, they are generally better tolerated in the long run and therefore are my first choice.

SSRIs can take two to four weeks or as long as eight weeks to be effective; they should be tapered off slowly to minimize withdrawal symptoms and the return of OCD behaviors.

## OTHER TREATMENTS

**Calming therapies** such as progressive relaxation, abdominal breathing, yoga, meditation, and regular aerobic exercise are all helpful in dealing with OCD symptoms. Hilda, who was stuck in her grocery store circuit, particularly benefited from brisk walks each morning and weekly classes that taught her how to breathe and meditate to calm her mind.

# PROBLEMS THAT CAN MIMIC OR COEXIST WITH OCD

**Hypochondriacs** are also saddled with obsessive thoughts of illness, but they usually aren't able to recognize that their obsessions are unreasonable, nor do they engage in compulsive actions.

**Tic disorders,** such as Tourette's syndrome, which features tics and uncontrollable vocalizations, resemble OCD and may coexist with it.

**Compulsive nail biting, skin picking, and hair pulling** (trichotillomania) have similarities to OCD, though it is unclear exactly how they are related.

**Impulse control problems,** such as compulsive gambling and anorexia nervosa, share features of OCD. However, since they're centered on only one activity, they are not usually considered to be a generalized problem like OCD.

**Depression.** Studies show that a majority of OCD sufferers have also undergone at least one episode of major depression in their lives. Some experts believe OCD causes the depression, while others think that depression and OCD only tend to coexist.

**Developmental disorders,** such as Asperger's syndrome or autism, include compulsive behaviors similar to OCD symptoms.

| Questions to Ask Your Parent If You Suspect OCD |
| --- |

■ Have you been having difficulty with daily activities, involving procrastination, indecision, or perfectionism?

■ Do you need to perform certain acts a number of times?

■ Do disturbing urges or images pop into your head?

■ Do you frequently engage in "what if" thinking: What if I didn't turn off the gas, lock the door, clean my hands well enough?

■ Do odd phrases or nonsensical words enter your mind?

■ Do you ever imagine that you have harmed yourself or someone else?

■ Do you feel compelled to confess or admit things?

■ Do you find that you need for things to be arranged in a certain orderly pattern?

■ Do you find yourself checking things over and over?

## HOW YOU CAN HELP

**Provide information and education.** Helping a parent realize that there is treatment that can control—if not cure—OCD symptoms is one of the chief ways an adult child can help. Without treatment, the prognosis for this disorder is not hopeful. Symptoms may wax and wane, but they rarely go away on their own.

**Make sure you differentiate** between personality type and full-blown disorder; a perfectionist mother does not necessarily have OCD.

**Be patient.** Don't tell a parent simply to stop his troublesome behaviors. Since he knows he can't do this through simple willpower, such requests will only serve to alienate him.

**Be positive and praise treatment efforts.** Since failure to comply with daily treatment regimens is common among the elderly, encourage consistency of medication or CBT. Let a parent know that OCD is a difficult condition to overcome without consistent treatment; reinforce that if a parent is determined to work hard, the prognosis is good.

**Ask for assistance.** Due to the secrecy and resistance of some OCD sufferers, you may need to have a primary-care doctor or a mediating therapist make a treatment referral for your parent.

**Arrange a family meeting.** Make sure all members of the immediate family are on the same page. The support of family and friends can make a big difference in the long-term success of OCD treatment.

**Find help for yourself.** It can be overwhelming to deal with the intensity and obstinance of a parent's OCD behavior. Finding a support group that includes others in the same position can be extremely helpful.

## SYMPTOMS OF OBSESSIVE-COMPULSIVE DISORDER

| PHYSIOLOGICAL | BEHAVIORAL | COGNITIVE |
|---|---|---|
| Marked distress if obsessions/compulsions are blocked | Repetitive, persistent behaviors (counting, checking, washing) that relieve anxiety briefly | Repetitive, intrusive, persistent thoughts that are recognized as unnecessary and inappropriate |

# 7

# POSTTRAUMATIC STRESS DISORDER

## SIGNS YOUR PARENT MAY HAVE POSTTRAUMATIC STRESS DISORDER

- Frequent nightmares or flashbacks about a traumatic past event, such as a combat incident, natural disaster, assault, accident, or sexual violation
- Morbid fixation on this event
- Sudden acute fearfulness
- Easily startled
- Overly vigilant about personal safety
- Can't concentrate or relax
- Sleeplessness and fatigue
- Persistent irritability
- Difficulty handling pressure or stress
- Self-medicates with alcohol or drugs
- Hypersensitivity
- Emotional detachment and lack of interest

What do you do when a battle your father fought in forty-five years ago becomes the dominant preoccupation of his life? Or your mother begins re-living details of a deadly car crash she once witnessed?

What is an appropriate response for a parent who has survived a violent assault or endured the horrors of a concentration camp?

Horror, disbelief, fear, grief, guilt—these are some of the ways we are hardwired as humans to react to trauma. It is natural for survivors of violence to respond to horrific events with a series of psychological responses that range from helplessness to intense fear. Yet even when faced with the most horrific tragedies, most people eventually heal and are able to move past these emotions.

But patients suffering from posttraumatic stress disorder (PTSD) are not able to progress past these events. The traumatic stressor becomes the centerpiece of their psyche, the dominant force in their lives. PTSD can become a debilitating, persistent condition in which sufferers are preoccupied and tormented with frightening memories of their ordeals—sometimes even reliving them.

Unlike other anxiety disorders, PTSD is *always* based on an identifiable cause. In fact, a diagnosis of PTSD requires that a patient has met a "stressor criterion"—exposure to an event that is considered traumatic. This is most often an event involving death or injury; for example, a plane crash that a patient was involved in—or a plane crash that she witnessed. This trauma is then relived through nightmares, flashbacks, and symptoms such as sleeplessness that persist over time.

A triggering event can be recent or it can be far in the past, as with an elderly former infantryman who suddenly finds himself having flashbacks to battle scenes.

This was the case with Sam, a glider pilot who'd survived the invasion of Normandy during World War II, but lost many of his friends during the attack. Sam was nineteen at the time of the invasion and returned home soon after to a hero's welcome. He quickly put his war experiences behind him and concentrated on starting a business and a large family. He avoided talking about his war years with his wife or children and refused to watch TV programs or movies related to that time.

He kept his life filled with activity. He was a deacon in the church and became the owner of a chain of automobile dealerships in New Jersey, working long hours and eventually amassing a small fortune.

After his retirement and the sudden death of his wife, Sam's eldest daughter, Sara, noticed an abrupt change in her father. He began having frequent nightmares and getting up in the middle of the night to call her.

"At first I thought it was grief over my mother," Sara said. "But these nightmares always centered on the war and his old compatriots. He talked about them by name—I couldn't hang up on him once he started."

At the same time Sam began experiencing spells of anxiety during the day—he broke out in a sweat whenever he heard loud noises, such as a car backfiring, thinking it was a gunshot. He also developed an overconcern with physical safety, installing burglar alarms in his house and displaying a sudden distrust of strangers. One afternoon, while he was driving his granddaughter to a dance class, a plane passed close overhead, and Sam pulled over to the side of the road and broke into sobs.

This was the point when Sam came to see me, and we began to explore how his past and present seemed to have dovetailed with this disorder. It was not so much that Sam had not previously dealt with the painfulness of his past life, but that the ways he had learned to cope—by keeping busy at his job and constructing a shield around himself and his family—had suddenly disappeared and left him vulnerable to a tendency he'd had all along.

The longer we live, the more traumatic events we experience or witness—from accidents to combat to violent crime. By late life, we have become compilations not only of pleasurable memories, but sorrows and losses. And the older we are, the more physically vulnerable we become to attacks and mishaps, which may result in deeper, more long-lasting results.

In this chapter, I will deal with sufferers like Sam, who are assailed by memories of traumas, both recent and far in the past.

# PTSD SYMPTOMS

PTSD generally has four broad symptoms:

### 1. An identifiable traumatic trigger.

This is something that the person is able to recognize and describe. This event isn't a secret or mystery—a parent can tell you that they were in a car crash or survived a hurricane or flood.

This trigger typically involves the experience or the witnessing of a traumatic event where death or threatened death was involved and where a parent felt helplessness or horror.

This can be a single traumatic event, such as a disaster or assault, or a number of smaller ones, such as repeated war battles, sexual abuse, or disaster scenes.

Research after the Oklahoma City bombing and the 9/11 attacks shows that between 5 and 20 percent of those exposed to such severe trauma continue to relive it and feel unable to get it out of their minds.[1] They have flashbacks, and disturbed sleep, and experience chronic worry and distress.

The exception to this identifiable trigger is in repressed memory syndrome. In this disorder, therapists elicit recovered memories, often involving sexual abuse, from patients who otherwise have no active remembrance, using techniques that have often been called into question; many of these recovered memories reports have later been found to be false.

### 2. Intrusive reexperiencing of a stressful event.

In PTSD, the memory of an event, or an actual image of it, pops into a person's head or intrudes into his consciousness. This flashback is usually vivid, irresistible, and not controllable. He may also experience a reliving of the experience through nightmares.

A component of this vivid reexperience is an accompanying emotional state—tension, fear, and distress—the very feelings a parent may have felt at the time of the original event. Because of these reactions, a sufferer may also have difficulties maintaining work and social relationships.

**3. Avoidance or an attempt to resist similar situations or triggers associated with the original event.**

A patient who experienced a battlefield trauma involving planes or helicopters might feel unable to go near an airport for fear of triggering fearful memories.

This is unlike a phobia, where a patient says, "It's silly but I'm just scared to fly." Instead, a PTSD sufferer might say: "If I go to an airport and hear those engines, I know it's going to trigger memories of the battlefield, and I'm going to experience terrible fear."

Another manifestation of avoidance in PTSD occurs when a sufferer cuts himself off from experiencing strong emotions and seems to become physically and emotionally numb.

**4. Hyperarousal.**

These symptoms can include insomnia, chronic fatigue, persistent irritability, violent outbursts, a constant state of alert, and increased startle response.

## AN ANCIENT DISORDER

While the term "PTSD" has been in common usage only for the last twenty years, the fact that people exposed to overwhelming trauma can be troubled and tormented for the rest of their lives has long been recognized. The psychic wounds of war, in particular, have been noted since antiquity. Descriptions of battle trauma go back to the ancient Greeks, who described warriors who never psychologically recovered from their inner wounds.

Post-combat syndromes include a wide variety of symptoms, ranging from fatigue and depression to respiratory and cardiovascular problems. Depending upon the conflict, these symptoms can be attributed to the psychological stress of military action, physical exertion, or illness.

Each war has its own name for this syndrome. It was called "shell shock" in World War I, from the trench warfare that was common; in World War II it was called "combat fatigue"; in the Civil War, "soldier's heart." Today it's called "combat stress reaction." Symptoms seem to differ from one conflict to the next. In World War I, British soldiers' health complaints centered on the heart, while in World War II, stomach difficulties were more common.[2]

Children of vets from World War II, Korea, and Vietnam are often surprised to discover that PTSD can occur in a parent decades after a traumatic event.

"How could my dad develop this after almost fifty years have passed?" Sam's son asked me.

Yet it's not uncommon, in the delayed form of PTSD, for symptoms to appear years after the trauma. In Sam's case, his hero's welcome and swift reentry into a post–World War II economy enabled him to push disturbing thoughts out of his mind. It was only later, after the isolation of retirement and the stress of his widowhood, that these issues resurfaced.

Sam's son, a Vietnam vet, experienced a much different welcome when he returned from his war, as well as being subjected to different stressors, such as environmental agents while in combat, but he never developed PTSD himself. In fact, there are many individuals who suffer crushing traumas and, after a period of sorrow, go on to rebuild their lives.

So what predicts who develops PTSD and who doesn't?

## WHAT PREDICTS PTSD?

### TEMPERAMENT

People with personality traits that include the tendency to worry and become anxious in the face of upsetting events are more likely to develop PTSD than those who are even-tempered.

People possess varying thresholds for trauma. What is felt as horrific by one person may barely faze another. That PTSD occurs in only a subset of those exposed to trauma suggests that risk may be influenced by individual differences that may be at least somewhat inherited.

A number of twin studies indicate genetic influences on PTSD symptoms and vulnerabilities. Genetic differences also seem to influence the exposure to certain traumas; this might be due to personality differences that influence environmental choices.[3]

## Severity of Event, Proximity, and Length of Exposure

There is a difference between being involved in—or witnessing—a fender bender and being in the middle of a horrific car accident that involves loss of life. When it comes to developing PTSD, the severity of the trauma plays a significant role.

Proximity to the traumatic event is another PTSD predictor. During the Mount St. Helens volcanic eruption, a mountainside collapsed into a nearby river, causing a thirty-foot tidal wave that drowned a number of people who lived in the valley.[4] Studies showed that those who lived closer to the river were more likely to develop lasting PTSD symptoms, even if they weren't actually hurt.

Since World War II, other studies have also shown that the more prolonged the exposure to the battlefront, the higher the likelihood of developing PTSD.[5] Exposure of two to three months dramatically increased the likelihood of a soldier developing PTSD symptoms. Since World War II and Korea, this has been taken into account by the armed services, who now rotate people away from the front.

## Traumatic Early Experiences

Early-life exposure to terrible stress—sexual abuse, abandonment, growing up in an environment of violence—increases the likelihood of developing PTSD. In fact, research shows that severe trauma or stress can cause lasting damage to the brain, specifically the hippocampus, which is often found to be smaller in size. One theory is that the hippocampus is particularly sensitive to cortisol, a stress hormone that exists in excess in severe PTSD sufferers. Another theory, based on studies of identical twins, in which one twin experienced trauma and the other did not, is that a small hippocampus suggests a genetic predisposition to PTSD, rather than stress being the cause.[6]

## NORMAL RESPONSE OR DISORDER?

After a trauma, it's perfectly natural for people to experience anxiety symptoms for days or weeks. These are a sign of PTSD only when they are present for more than a month, cause continuing distress, and become intrusive, as in the following case.

Phyllis worked at a stressful profession, as a 911 operator in Connecticut, and had suffered throughout her life from a fretful, overly anxious temperament. She'd commuted to her job for thirty years along the same stretch of Route I-95 near New Haven, always driving safely in the slow lane and never passing other cars.

But one December morning, her careful driving could not protect her. A layer of ice had created hazardous highway conditions, and she was involved in a serious ten-car pileup. Several drivers were thrown from their cars, and mangled wreckage was everywhere. There were a number of casualties, including a child, whom Phyllis witnessed being pulled from the rubble. Phyllis was at the end of the pileup and only sustained light injuries to her arm and wrist, but she was airlifted with the rest of the victims to the hospital where she was released the next day.

The trauma Phyllis had suffered wasn't evident to anyone but her family. In the days that followed, they noted a marked difference in her behavior and demeanor. She was irritable, had difficulty sleeping, and experienced frequent flashbacks to the accident. She also developed a rapid heartbeat, became easily startled, and refused to get in a car as a driver or passenger.

This accident seemed to validate and accentuate the anxiety she'd felt all her life.

"It was as if she'd always expected something like this to happen," her husband said. "We kept telling her that she was lucky to be alive, but she was miserable and anxious anyhow."

Several months after the accident, Phyllis decided to take early retirement, because she no longer felt comfortable commuting. Once home, alone and unoccupied, her symptoms increased. When her daughter visited from out of town, she was shocked to find a new version of her mother—a fearful, essentially homebound woman who could talk of little other than the accident she had been in nearly six months before. This was coupled with a cool, "numb" demeanor that her daughter found particularly shocking.

"She pulled away from all of us, even her grandkids. She didn't laugh; she didn't cry. She was like a zombie."

This psychic numbing is a common feature of PTSD sufferers, who are no longer able to handle deep feelings or strong emotions.

It was at this point that her daughter insisted on bringing Phyllis to see me.

A parent like Phyllis, who is already anxious, may be more vulnerable to trauma and have more difficulty coping. Phyllis's temperament along with the isolation and boredom she experienced after quitting her job, all probably contributed to her PTSD.

In Otis's case, it wasn't one traumatic experience but a whole career of them that hit him upon retirement. A fireman for forty years, Otis regularly witnessed scenes of devastation. But it wasn't until he retired and relocated with his son and family to Florida that he began exhibiting classic PTSD symptoms. He had vivid dreams and reexperienced certain fire scenes where he'd seen people perish. He broke out in sweat whenever he heard a siren; or as his son put it, "he tranced out for a few minutes" as if he were back at a fire scene.

Otis grew increasingly jumpy and irritable, rarely leaving the house. His dreams were so terrifying that he sat up all night, and then he began bringing a bottle of bourbon into his bedroom.

It took several months before his son realized that his father had a serious problem—and then several months more to convince him to seek help.

The son said, "I know other old-timers like Dad who get worked up whenever there's a fireman's funeral or it's the anniversary of a big fire. I guess I thought it was normal, just an occupational hazard. But I finally had to face the fact that Dad's problem was bigger than that. It was affecting him all the time. He couldn't watch TV or even get in the car. He was so afraid of hearing a siren or seeing a fire."

# TREATMENT

## Psychotherapeutic Techniques

### *Best Bets*

In my experience, practicing avoidance isn't beneficial for those who have been exposed to a traumatic stressor; it's far better for a patient to banish a trauma by finding a way to face it. That's why I find **cognitive-behavior therapy** the most helpful for PTSD sufferers.

The basic thrust of cognitive therapy is that sufferers have learned maladaptive ways of thinking that contribute to their anxiety. Cognitive-therapy techniques teach patients to evaluate their irrational fears and negative beliefs and come up with other ways of dealing with them.

One way is to banish the negative self-talk that often feeds into PTSD symptoms and encourages avoidance. After her accident, my patient Phyllis told herself that driving was treacherous and that she could never do it again. She cut herself off from all outside activities, which further encouraged her escalating feelings of fragility and strengthened her PTSD.

One way to combat her entrenched habit of expecting the worst was to question the validity of her negative perception: "Highway driving is now always treacherous for me." I countered this negative statement with facts. In Phyllis's case, she had driven to work for over thirty years without so much as a fender bender. In fact, her driving record was without a single black mark in all her years of commuting. Furthermore, the accident she was involved in was caused by another driver and affected by road conditions over which she had no control.

So if Phyllis looked at the whole picture, she could say: "The evidence from years of driving is that highway travel isn't dangerous. I have not had a single accident or ticket after commuting to work five days a week for over thirty years." This kind of work takes practice, but it can be highly effective.

Another method, called **thought-stopping,** can help a patient with negative thoughts. Otis used this technique whenever he found himself ruminating about a fire. He wore an elastic band around his wrist and said aloud

"No! Stop it!" and snapped the band whenever unwanted thoughts began intruding into his mind.

Behavior approaches include exposure, where a patient faces his trauma by either imagining it in detail or by visiting places that are strong reminders.

In some cases, traumas can be confronted all at once, using a method called **flooding.** But in most cases, it is preferable to work gradually up to the trauma by using relaxation techniques and building up to it one increment at a time, using a method called **gradual exposure** or **desensitization.**

A goal for a parent such as Phyllis, who was so traumatized by her auto accident that she suffered flashbacks and wouldn't get back into a car, could be to eventually have her drive on the highway where the traumatic accident occurred. To prepare her for this, a therapist might use imagery techniques, where Phyllis systematically visualized herself in a calm place, then worked herself up in graded steps to finally seeing herself calmly driving on the feared highway.

Gradual desensitization would involve her taking incremental, real-life steps to the actual driving—such as driving on similar roads for short, then longer, periods with a support person, and being driven to the feared highway by a support person. The ultimate goal would be for her to drive to this location herself.

The idea behind this therapy is that while it may be helpful to talk about a trauma, it's better for a patient like Phyllis to actually start *driving* again.

## Other Nondrug Treatments

**Group therapy** is often recommended as a helpful adjunct to medication in PTSD, but I find this type of therapy isn't always the best route. PTSD sufferers are stuck in destructive-behavior cycles and maladaptive ways of thinking. Group therapy usually focuses on emotional support, but people with PTSD often need more than sympathy from peers—they need to change the way they're thinking and approaching their problems.

For an older parent such as Sam, however, who was anxious to share his trauma, finding a survivors' group where he could confide in others who have undergone similar events was a relief. The empathy provided by a group environment helped him confront the past and work through feelings of anxiety and grief.

Supportive **psychotherapy** can be beneficial for PTSD sufferers, helping a parent face his trauma in a safe environment. In talk therapy, a parent can gain new coping skills and learn to identify triggering life situations that might cause future difficulties or set off traumatic memories. The goal of this kind of therapy is to assist a parent in coping with stressful memories without being emotionally overwhelmed. It can also help to work through the feelings of fear and guilt that are so common. Hypnosis is sometimes used to have a survivor revisit the original trauma.

**Calming techniques,** such as deep breathing, visualization, and progressive relaxation can be beneficial for PTSD sufferers. In visualization techniques, patients train themselves to recall and visualize a particularly peaceful or pleasant place or situation whenever thoughts of the trauma occur. Deep abdominal breathing can also help calm PTSD symptoms.

**Physical exercise** has been shown to be helpful in alleviating PTSD symptoms. A recent study of Gulf War vets found that a combination of cognitive-behavior therapy and aerobic exercise provided relief for a number of PTSD symptoms, such as persistent pain and fatigue.[7]

## PHARMACOLOGICAL TREATMENTS

### Best Bets

Because of their tolerability and wide effectiveness and potency for a range of symptoms, **SSRIs** are my first choice for PTSD symptoms. SSRIs help restore the balance of the brain chemical serotonin, which reduces the symptoms of anxiety and depression. These drugs also have less serious side effects (nausea, insomnia, and sexual dysfunction) than older drugs, and fewer withdrawal problems.

Zoloft is the SSRI specifically approved by the FDA for PTSD treatment, but Paxil, Prozac, Celexa, and Luvox have also shown effectiveness. Effexor, which boosts both norepinephrine and serotonin, has also been used.

Parents should be reminded that they may feel better in as little as two weeks, but that it can take four to eight weeks for the full effects of an SSRI to be felt. Depending upon the drug, many side effects abate after the first few weeks of treatment. If one SSRI is not effective, another may be. These medications should be tapered off slowly, under a doctor's supervision.

## Other Choices

**Benzodiazepines** such as Valium, Xanax, and Ativan are fast-acting antianxiety agents that should be used only short-term for the elderly, or until other drugs, such as SSRIs, take effect. I almost never prescribe them for PTSD, since the symptoms are usually long-standing.

These medications should be reserved for limited interventions due to their addictive properties, the possibility of overdose, and their troublesome side effects, which include sedation and psychomotor impairment. If a benzodiazepine has been used for any extended period, the dosage should be tapered off gradually.

While studies have proven the effectiveness of **tricyclics** such as Pamelor, Elavil, and Tofranil for PTSD, they should only be used as a last resort. Elavil and Tofranil in particular should be avoided in older adults because of their many side effects, especially memory impairment, increased heart rate, daytime drowsiness, dizziness, and a high overdose risk.

# PROBLEMS THAT CAN MIMIC OR COEXIST WITH PTSD

### Survivor's guilt

It is not uncommon for those who survive a disaster to experience a period when they feel guilt that they lived while others died. These feelings usually pass and don't manifest in the reexperiencing of the trauma, as in PTSD.

### Panic disorder

In both panic disorder and PTSD, a parent may show great resistance to a feared activity, such as flying. But unlike PTSD, with panic disorder there is not necessarily a precipitating trauma that causes this reaction.

### Agoraphobia

A PTSD sufferer who is trying to "avoid" traumatic reminders may be afraid to leave the house, and may develop agoraphobia as a result.

### Dissociative and personality disorders

These may result in a variety of difficult behaviors, including rage and impulsiveness. Sufferers aren't as eager to avoid triggers as in PTSD, and have had lifelong interpersonal difficulties.

### Substance abuse and alcohol abuse

PTSD symptoms may be masked by self-medication and alcohol use. Some experts suggest that these issues be addressed at the same time as PTSD treatment.

### Depression

This is often a component of PTSD, either as a cause or an effect. If the depression is caused by the PTSD, it may be alleviated once the disorder is treated; if not, it needs to be treated separately.

## Questions to Ask Your Parent If You Suspect PTSD

■ Have you been having recurring dreams or intrusive recollections about a traumatic event in the past?

■ Are you avoiding activities that are related to this traumatic event?

■ Are you experiencing fatigue and difficulty falling asleep?

■ Are you having difficulty handling stressful situations?

*(continued)*

■ Is it hard for you to concentrate or sit still?

■ Are you feeling short-fused, or irritated at small things?

■ Do you feel a heightened sense of alertness?

■ Do you feel physically or emotionally numb?

## HOW YOU CAN HELP

**Make sure you get the correct diagnosis.** It's important to differentiate PTSD from feelings of grief and loss that normally result from a traumatic event. Symptoms must be persistent and life-altering. Just because your dad becomes weepy whenever he talks about an old infantry battle doesn't necessarily mean he has PTSD.

**Get info.** The Department of Veterans Affairs and crisis clinics for victims of assault and abuse have information that can be helpful for sufferers of PTSD symptoms. There are also many books that can help guide survivors in the process of recovery. However, some of these resources claim that everyone exposed to traumatic events should receive treatment, a statement that is often untrue. Others overemphasize the importance of talking about feelings and downplay the importance of changing behavior.

**Find support groups** where trauma survivors can learn new behaviors. Psychoeducation and group interaction can also help relieve irrational feelings of guilt. But most eventually help people *lessen* their focus on emotions and increase their focus on positive change.

**Make sure a parent is getting enough sleep.** Lack of sleep is a common symptom of PTSD, one that can exacerbate symptoms. Fatigue can be especially troublesome for these sufferers, since their dreams may be even more troublesome than their daytime thoughts. If your parent isn't getting enough sleep, make sure you tell the doctor; drugs such as Ambien and Trazodone are often recommended.

**Be on the lookout for substance abuse** and increased alcohol usage. Heavy drinking is often used by PTSD sufferers to dull their pain and distress and sometimes to facilitate sleep. This can be particularly dangerous when mixed with medication.

**Foster connection.** While drugs and therapy can often treat this trauma, Dr. Jonathan Shay, who treats the spiritual injuries of combat, believes that other components—connection and trust—are just as essential. Because of this, he refers his patients to arts programs and religious congregations in addition to therapy.[8]

## SYMPTOMS OF POSTTRAUMATIC STRESS DISORDER

| PHYSIOLOGICAL | BEHAVIORAL | COGNITIVE |
|---|---|---|
| Poor sleep | Avoidance of triggers | Recurrent, distressing recollections or dreams about a specific event |
| Hypervigilance and alertness (i.e., heightened startle) | Impaired social or work performance | |

# 8

# PANIC DISORDER

## SIGNS YOUR PARENT MAY HAVE A PANIC DISORDER

- Frequent spells of intense apprehension and fear
- Physical symptoms, such as chest pain, difficulty breathing, sweating, dizziness, nausea
- Believes is suffering from a life-threatening disease, even though physical exams are normal
- Has attacks that appear out of the blue, or result from exposure to a dreaded situation
- Exhibits unwillingness to engage in activities that involve going out or being in high or closed spaces, such as crossing a bridge, riding an escalator, boarding a bus or plane, or going food shopping
- Fear of dying, losing control, or being publicly humiliated if confronted by fearful activity
- Limiting and self-restricting activities in order to avoid these attacks
- Waking in the night with a feeling of terror

In panic, more than any other disorder, an older parent is likely to experience frightening physical symptoms such as shortness of breath, trembling, numbness, and chest pain that may convince her—and you—that she has a life-threatening medical condition.

With generalized anxiety disorder, a parent worries that she's physically ill. With a panic disorder, she physically *feels* that she is. And it's often the fear of an attack—the *anticipatory anxiety*—that precipitates another, causing a self-perpetuating cycle that is impossible to break without treatment.

It can be frightening and frustrating to deal with a parent who suffers from attacks that include such dire physical symptoms as chest pain and difficulty breathing, but who, according to doctors, is healthy.

But it is even more terrifying to *be* a sufferer, such as Elizabeth, who frantically shuttled from one emergency room to another, convinced she was dying from an undiagnosed malady that no one else took seriously.

"What do you say to your mother when she's crumpled up on the couch, gasping for breath—'No, you're not really having trouble breathing'?" her daughter asked me. "I could tell by her face that she sincerely was, but no one could explain it."

Her mother, seventy-five-year-old Elizabeth, had always been an independent woman and had lived on her own in a Manhattan apartment since her husband's death years before. In the last months, Elizabeth reported to her daughter that she'd begun having "spells" during which she experienced difficulty breathing, a sensation of being smothered, and a rush of heat and disorientation.

Her daughter, terrified by these accounts, instructed her mother to call the ambulance whenever she had such an attack. But this advice seemed only to accelerate Elizabeth's panic. In the next weeks, she made half a dozen trips to the emergency room, where she was initially given oxygen for hyperventilation—or rapid breathing—a common feature of panic attacks. But the oxygen was quickly stopped when the doctor decided that her problem was "psychological."

By the time Elizabeth and her daughter arrived in my office, I found two fretful women—the daughter nearly as distraught as her mother—with a pile of negative reports from the emergency room.

When I talked to Elizabeth about how and when these attacks occurred, she revealed that they almost always happened on the weekend, on a crowded street where she was dropped off by a senior-center bus. This new stop in an unfamiliar neighborhood seemed to trigger her discomfort. But she also told me that she'd had similar attacks before—especially during the illness of her husband—that she'd never told anyone about. "I was scared that they meant I was losing my mind or getting Alzheimer's," she admitted. She also reported that her blood pressure medicine had recently been changed and the dosage increased.

I strongly suspected that Elizabeth was suffering from a panic disorder, and a full physical workup and drug evaluation proved this to be true.

This chapter will look at how panic can be accentuated and complicated by a number of late-life concerns, including increased physical maladies and frailties, and stressful life events.

## LOSING CONTROL

Panic disorders are commonly heralded by a sudden assault of intense fear during which a parent feels apprehension, along with a variety of physical symptoms, including difficulty breathing, chest tightness and pain, rapid or erratic heartbeat, tingling around the lips, nausea, trembling, and shaking.

This combination of fear and physical symptoms can cause a person to feel such panic that he wants to flee the situation for fear he might otherwise collapse or even die. This sense of losing control, while a common symptom of a panic attack, may also be a reality in the lives of some elderly parents, who find their independence and mobility curtailed. These sufferers may cut themselves off from others and hide their symptoms, resulting in further isolation and depression.

Panic episodes usually peak in ten minutes and occur with variable frequency, sometimes several times a day or every few weeks. They can occur for no apparent reason or be triggered by an event, such as going over a bridge, boarding a plane, or simply the anticipation of these events. In late life, the panic trigger may be more benign, as with Elizabeth, whose attacks were triggered by an unfamiliar neighborhood. While the prevalence of panic in the elderly is less than 1 percent, the disorder occurs in females more often than males and often begins in early life.[1]

## ILLNESS OR PANIC?

The symptoms of panic disorder resemble a number of life-threatening illnesses, including heart and lung disease, epilepsy, asthma, and thyroid problems. The existence of physical symptoms makes this disorder a diagnostic challenge with seniors, who are more likely to suffer from a wider range of serious conditions. Many sufferers cycle through a variety of doctors and emergency room visits without being properly diagnosed.

It's important to remember that it's not unusual or abnormal for a parent to have an attack of panic after a stressful or upsetting situation. When Russell was first diagnosed with cancer, he underwent a period when he had intense spells of panic, trembling, and dizziness.

"I didn't understand what was happening to me," he said. "I felt like my whole life was falling apart."

However, Russell's attacks abated after a few weeks, once his treatment plan was stabilized and he became more knowledgeable about the course of his particular disease—and hopeful about his chances of recovery. His panic was situational and short-lived.

With a panic *disorder,* on the other hand, attacks are persistent, last at least half an hour, and often come out of the blue. While they may be precipitated by a situational trigger, it is the *panic attack itself* that often becomes the dreaded event.

Some sufferers, such as Edna, can pinpoint the event that precipitated their first attack.

Edna had her first experience of panic at age sixty-two, when a train she was traveling in derailed. Even though she only suffered a minor ankle sprain, she developed difficulty breathing and chest tightness, and was taken to the emergency room of a local hospital, where she was given a dose of Xanax and released.

She experienced another attack later that summer after she nearly had a car accident. As a result of these two incidents, she began to dread the resurgence of her panic symptoms and lay sleepless with a feeling of impending doom. Eventually, she began experiencing regular bouts of chest tightness and breathing difficulty.

These symptoms so preoccupied her that she started going from one doctor to another. Over time, she underwent overlapping series of EKGs, lung X-rays, stress tests, ultrasounds, and CAT scans—and always received a clean bill of health.

Yet none of these results comforted her for long. As she told me: "How can I be healthy when I feel so bad?"

After several months of this regimen, Edna began to worry that she was developing dementia, something she admitted only later to her daughter. "The doctors said it was nothing. I knew it was. Their denying it only made my panic worse. I'm sure they thought I was just a crazy old lady who wanted attention."

Her daughter said: "By the time I put together what was happening, I found that Mom had been to over a dozen doctors and had every diagnostic test under the sun. Four EKGs in different emergency rooms . . . Nothing was coordinated. I had no idea she was going through all this alone."

Unfortunately, there are cases when a parent's physical symptoms may be checked, rechecked, and ultimately dismissed without anyone realizing that she is legitimately suffering from a real disorder and that it's panic.

In cases such as Edna's, coordinating doctor visits and monitoring consistency of care and treatment are some of the most important acts an adult child can perform.

## WHAT CAUSES PANIC?

### GENES AND PANIC

While the causes of panic disorder are still not entirely clear, family and twin studies indicate this disorder has a strong genetic component. Nearly half of those suffering from panic have at least one affected relative.[2] In fact, having a close relative with panic disorder is the most commonly noted risk factor in newly diagnosed patients. What seems to be inherited is an abnormally sensitive "fear circuit" in the brain.

## $CO_2$ SENSITIVITY

Those who develop panic attacks are often overly sensitive to carbon dioxide ($CO_2$). Normally, increasing $CO_2$ levels in the body triggers an increased rate of breathing. During a panic attack, the brain sends a false suffocation alarm, signaling a shortage of oxygen or an increase in carbon dioxide. This results in the hyperventilation—or rapid breathing—that is a common symptom of panic attacks. In fact, a spontaneous attack can be induced by having a sufferer breathe carbon dioxide. Along with shortness of breath, symptoms of hyperventilation include tingling in the hands, feet, or lips; trembling; lightheadedness; and dizziness.

## NEUROBIOLOGY

Recent research indicates that those with panic disorder suffer from significant reductions of a serotonin receptor, 5 $HT1_A$, in several brain areas. Researchers used brain scans of people with panic to locate areas near the center of the brain with low numbers of serotonin receptors. They found that subjects with panic averaged a third fewer receptors in three different brain areas. These findings lend weight to the belief that panic disorder is caused by a specific brain abnormality. It's also likely that these receptor deficiencies are at least partly genetic.[3]

MRIs have also shown a number of structural brain abnormalities, primarily in the temporal lobe, in those who suffer from panic disorders.[4]

## MEDICAL CONDITIONS

Certain medical conditions, such as hyperthyroidism, mitral valve prolapse, and reactions to sedatives and tranquilizers, can cause or make panic worse.

For seniors who do not eat an adequate diet, blood sugar may fall too low and cause panic-like symptoms. Hypoglycemia can be the cause of panic attacks or make preexisting ones worse.

## TRAUMA

A traumatic event is often a factor in triggering a person's initial panic attack, which may then develop into a disorder. Edna's train derailment earlier in her life is a good example of this.

Common precipitative traumas include the death of a spouse, a serious illness, or a major change, such as moving from a lifelong home into a retirement community.

# TREATMENT

## PSYCHOTHERAPEUTIC TECHNIQUES

### *Best Bets*

**Cognitive-behavior therapy** is an effective intervention for panic disorders in the elderly, especially in treating the dysfunctional thought processes that generate and maintain anxiety and in extinguishing conditioned fear responses.

Many parents suffering from panic tend to misinterpret bodily sensations as indications of an oncoming attack. They say to themselves: "My heart's beating too fast. What if I'm dying?" Such anxious self-dialogue can actually precipitate attacks and make them worse.

By changing the way sufferers think about their panic symptoms, and how they behave regarding them, CBT can help them handle and reinterpret symptoms in a more rational way.

A calming coping statement, such as "I accept this feeling. It's only adrenaline in my system; it won't kill me," might be used to replace a patient's typical panicked thoughts.

Behavioral techniques such as gradual exposure to more adaptive situations, breathing retraining, and development of anxiety-management skills are also beneficial. Using these techniques, Elizabeth learned to watch her symptoms instead of immediately reacting to them and thereby making herself even more terrified. She used abdominal breathing and progressive muscle relaxation to calm herself at the onset of an attack instead of automatically calling the ambulance for another futile trip to the emergency room.

She also learned to distract herself from negative preoccupations by thought-stopping—saying "No!" to herself whenever she found herself drifting into panic. She also used other diversionary techniques, such as taking a brisk walk or calling a friend.

## OTHER NONDRUG TREATMENTS

**Calming and relaxation techniques** such as visualization, hypnosis, abdominal breathing, meditation, and yoga are often effective adjuncts to medical and psychological treatments.

These techniques can be used to help fend off panic if a patient is experiencing or anticipating situations that have triggered attacks in the past. The pounding heart, rapid breathing, sweating, and trembling that are common panic symptoms are the result of adrenaline release. If a patient learns to observe rather than react to these symptoms, they eventually diminish as the adrenaline is reabsorbed.

A technique to ward off panic and hyperventilation involves deep abdominal breathing—inhaling slowly through the nose, holding the breath for a count of three, and exhaling slowly in a controlled manner through the mouth for a count of four.

Another method is progressive muscle relaxation, where muscle groups are systematically tightened, held, then slowly released. This actually teaches a person how to control and combat the sensation of muscle tightness and tension that is a part of panic.

Regular physical exercise is also a proven way to banish feelings of panic and to work off stress. Elizabeth found that a brisk daily walk and a weekly yoga class helped her ward off her attacks.

## PHARMACOLOGICAL TREATMENTS

### Best Bets

**Serotonin reuptake inhibitors (SSRIs),** which boost the neurotransmitter serotonin, are my first regimen of choice for this disorder, because they have powerful antipanic properties, are not addictive, typically require only one dose a day, and have milder and less serious side effects for the elderly than older drugs.

The SSRIs Paxil and Zoloft have been expressly approved for treatment of panic disorder, but others, such as Lexapro and Prozac, have also shown effectiveness.

Side effects that may occur from these drugs include diarrhea, weight gain, stomach upset, sexual dysfunction, and insomnia. Patients should be told that they may feel better in as little as two weeks, but that it can take up to eight for the full effects of an SSRI to be felt. Depending upon the drug, many side effects abate after the first few weeks of treatment.

If one SSRI doesn't work, or causes unpleasant side effects, another may be better tolerated. A patient should only discontinue these drugs under a doctor's supervision.

Drugs that combine the actions of SSRIs with blockage of norepinephrine reuptake such as Effexor are also effective in treating panic and are as beneficial as SSRIs. Side effects are similar to SSRIs, but in addition, Effexor can increase blood pressure.

## *Other Choices*

**Benzodiazepines** such as Xanax and Klonopin are effective drugs that are often prescribed for sudden onset panic attacks; Xanax has been FDA-approved for this purpose. Because they are fast-acting, these drugs are often used short-term for immediate relief or until SSRIs take effect.

However, these muscle relaxants and sleeping aids are problematic for long-term use in the elderly because of their addictiveness, withdrawal symptoms, and the possibility of abuse. Their side effects are more troublesome and include memory problems, unsteady walking, and drowsiness.

**Tricyclics** such as Pamelor, Tofranil, and Anafranil have a long history of use in panic disorders and may still be used when other treatments aren't effective. These drugs have a number of adverse side effects, including low blood pressure, abnormal heart rhythm, memory loss, constipation, and difficulty urinating. Because of their cardiac effects, these drugs should be used only when other medications have failed.

**MAOIs (monamine oxidase inhibitors)** such as Nardil and Parnate are another class of drugs effective for panic. The drawback with these medications is that they require dietary restrictions. A parent must adhere to a diet that omits a number of foods, including cheese, chocolate, aged meat, and wines, all of which contain tyramine, which can cause serious interactions. Since MAOIs also cause low blood pressure and weight gain, I use them only for elderly patients who have not responded to other medications.

## PROBLEMS THAT CAN MIMIC OR COEXIST WITH PANIC DISORDER

**Hyperventilation** often occurs with panic attacks, and can cause symptoms such as dizziness or fainting. Learning how to control hyperventilation can help a patient avoid future attacks.

**Serious medical conditions** share the same symptoms as panic disorder and must be ruled out before treatment can be started. Among the medical conditions that mimic the symptoms of panic are irregular heart rhythms, an overactive thyroid, some types of seizure disorder, and asthma.

**Mitral valve prolapse,** a cardiac condition involving the mitral valve of the heart, is more commonly associated in women with panic disorder. Whether the two conditions are genetically linked or the prolapse is a contributor to development of panic is not yet known.

**Diet.** Caffeine, nicotine, and low blood sugar can all cause shakiness and aggravate panic symptoms.

**Dementia,** a common cause of anxiety in late life, can eventually result in the development of panic. Early signs of memory loss and other cognitive impairments may cause a patient to become isolated and fearful and precipitate feelings of panic.

**Agoraphobia and phobia.** Panic attacks often cause sufferers to limit their lives to a safe zone, usually their houses or apartments, where attacks don't occur. This self-restriction of movement can result in agoraphobia, an inability to venture beyond safe surroundings because of intense fear. It's also common for people with panic disorder to develop phobias about places or situations where their attacks have occurred, such as supermarkets or everyday circumstances.

**Depression.** As with many anxiety disorders, people who are suffering from panic disorder are often depressed about their condition. In some cases, the panic may be causing the depression, and once the panic is treated the depression disappears. In other cases, the two problems simply coexist and must be treated separately.

**Substance abuse.** Alcohol dependence and drug use or withdrawal (particularly from benzodiazepines and barbiturates) may cause panic or be features of panic disorders. These substances, used to provide relief, create a vicious cycle, often accelerating anxiety and causing more panic.

## Questions to Ask Your Parent If You Suspect Panic Disorder

■ Have you been secretly worried over physical symptoms, such as shortness of breath or chest pain, that your doctor insists aren't related to illness?

■ Have you been making emergency-room visits or going to a number of different doctors for the same set of symptoms?

■ Do you feel as if you're going crazy because of these unexplained symptoms?

■ Have you been curtailing any of your normal activities because of these symptoms?

■ Are you combining different medications or drinking alcohol to make these symptoms go away?

■ Do you live in fear or dread of these attacks?

## HOW YOU CAN HELP

**Make sure your parent has a thorough diagnostic workup** to rule out life-threatening illnesses. Never assume that a parent with chest pain or difficulty breathing is suffering only from panic.

Standard laboratory tests that may be performed in a workup include a blood count; kidney, liver, and thyroid function tests; an electrocardiogram (EKG); and a test of blood electrolytes.

These tests should eliminate most of the more common medical conditions that can mimic panic disorder, such as cardiac and pulmonary disease, thyroid disorders, and liver problems.

**Help your parent keep medical records and coordinate treatment.** It is helpful for a parent to show test results to a doctor, psychiatrist, or counselor to facilitate diagnosis, and to avoid duplication of testing or medication.

**Once panic disorder has been diagnosed, be reassuring.** You might tell a mother who is in the middle of an attack: "I know it feels like you're dying, Mom, but remember what Dr. J. said. You're not ill. This is panic. You can't die from it."

**Ward off a hyperventilation attack** by having a parent breathe into a paper bag.

**Urge a parent not to self-medicate,** with alcohol or drugs, or to mix them.

**Offer your parent the following coping tips** to handle a panic attack:

- Release extra adrenaline by taking a brisk walk
- Take it easy, with deep, slow breaths
- Do a series of yoga stretches
- Accept the panic; don't judge it: observe it come and go
- Divert attention from symptoms by doing a crossword puzzle, gardening, or calling a friend
- Use positive self-talk, such as "It's only panic. It can't hurt me. I'll survive."

## SYMPTOMS OF PANIC DISORDER

| PHYSIOLOGICAL | BEHAVIORAL | COGNITIVE |
|---|---|---|
| Pounding heart | Avoidance of panic-inducing event | Feeling of unreality and losing control |
| Sweating | | |
| Nausea | | Fear of dying |
| Chest discomfort | | |
| Lightheadedness | | |
| Numbness and tingling | | |

# 9

# PHOBIA DISORDER

## SIGNS YOUR PARENT MAY HAVE A PHOBIA

- Demonstrates an unreasonable fear of a particular object or situation
- Avoids going into public unless accompanied by a close friend or relative
- Is overly sensitive to disapproval
- Avoids eating in public or attending social gatherings
- Demonstrates anxiety about entering closed-in spaces, such as elevators and tunnels, or traveling in vehicles
- Is easily embarrassed or ashamed
- Avoids eye contact
- Is fearful of any performance or public speech
- Blushes, trembles, and sweats when under scrutiny
- Worries about being able to escape
- Restricts activities to a minimum

Treating the unreasonable and persistent fears that are the hallmark of phobias can be challenging in the elderly, since leaving the house for a doctor's appointment, calling attention to one's symptoms, or even talking in public are the very kind of situations a phobic parent strives to avoid. In a sufferer's mind, a doctor visit may be viewed as a perilous social event, speaking aloud a terrifying performance, and discussing personal symptoms a way of provoking painful scrutiny.

Anticipating the terror that these anxiety-provoking situations may cause, phobic parents may go to great lengths to keep away from the focus of their fears—walking up dozens of stairs to avoid an elevator or taking a bus across country rather than fly. But these avoidant behaviors ultimately only make phobias worse.

Phobic disorders are among the most prevalent of old age—up to 12 percent according to some studies.[1] Agoraphobia ranks as late life's most common phobia. The distress these phobias cause can severely isolate, incapacitate, and interfere with the functioning of an elderly parent, and in some cases make them housebound.

A phobic, like seventy-one-year-old Beth, a retired librarian, often recognizes that her terrors are unreasonable, but that doesn't prevent her from feeling them. When she came to see me, Beth reported that she intellectually understood it was crazy that she was too terrified to sit in the bleachers to watch her granddaughter's dance recital. She knew that she'd be surrounded by family and that no one would allow her to fall. But whether it was foolish or not didn't matter. Her mind and body were registering otherwise.

As a young woman, Beth had been pushed off a banister and broken her shoulder and arm so severely that she could barely use it for several years. This accident had made her so fearful and avoidant of heights that even decades later, the mere topic made her break out in a sweat.

Beth admitted with a certain sorrow that her phobias had kept her from partaking in many events in her family's life. "I've missed high school graduations, family vacations in the mountains, and basketball games coached by my son. This thing has had hold of me all my life, but it's even stronger now that I'm older."

"We've tried everything, even bribing her," her daughter says. "But nothing works."

Cajoling, encouraging, or challenging a parent with phobias isn't effective, since phobias are strong disorders that usually can't be cured without treatment.

Avoidance is a way of coping with phobias, but it's not a way of curing them. It was only when Beth agreed to therapy that her cycle of extreme fear was eventually broken.

This chapter will discuss symptoms and manifestations of phobias in late life and strategies that can prevent them from limiting the life of an elderly parent.

## PHOBIC SYMPTOMS

Parents with phobias exhibit one or more of the following signs and symptoms that interfere with their ability to function:

- An excessive, disruptive, and persistent fear of a situation or object
- An overwhelming urge to avoid the object or situation or flee from it
- Physical anxiety reactions when confronted with the dreaded situation or object, including shortness of breath, racing or irregular heartbeat, trembling, sweating, blushing, muscle twitching
- An irrational and uncontrollable preoccupation with the feared stimulus

## TYPES OF PHOBIAS

There are three main kinds of phobias: specific fears, agoraphobia, and social phobia.

## Specific Phobias

These are the most common type of phobias, centering on fear or dread of a particular object or situation. In the elderly, common phobias are of closed spaces, heights, illness, and animals. But there are as many manifestations of specific phobias as there are people who experience them, as the following list shows:

*Alektorophobia*—fear of chickens
*Blennophobia*—fear of slime
*Caligynephobia*—fear of beautiful women
*Epistaxiophobia*—fear of nosebleeds
*Genuphobia*—fear of knees
*Ichthyophobia*—fear of fish
*Lachanophobia*—fear of vegetables
*Mageirocophobia*—fear of cooking
*Novercaphobia*—fear of your mother-in-law
*Pteronophobia*—fear of being tickled by feathers
*Siderophobia*—fear of stars
*Thalassophobia*—fear of the sea
*Uranophobia*—fear of heaven

Specific phobias may be precipitated by a traumatic event, such as a dog bite, or, in Beth's case, an accident. A parent becomes phobic when she begins to irrationally avoid a situation—such as refusing to go outdoors after a dog bite. However, there may be no trigger; it is perfectly possible for a patient to have a dog phobia without ever experiencing a negative event in the past.

With a specific phobia, the most innocuous-seeming situation can loom large for a patient, who may go to great lengths to keep it secret.

"It took me months to figure out that my mother wouldn't visit us in our new apartment because she was terrified of riding up in the elevator," a nurse told me. "She was embarrassed to admit it, and she kept saying, 'I know it's ridiculous.' But it wasn't ridiculous to me. Her fear was strong enough to keep her from visiting her grandkids. We found a geriatric psychiatrist and got help for her right away."

## AGORAPHOBIA

The word literally means "fear of open spaces," and the condition often manifests in the elderly in a terror of going to the supermarket or store, then accelerates into avoidance of any location outside a zone of safety—usually a parent's house or apartment. Like specific phobias, this disorder can be the result of a panic attack triggered by a specific trauma—for example, a fall in a supermarket, which initiates a panic attack and then progresses to a general terror of going shopping again.

Or it may be that a person has always experienced these sorts of difficulties, but the stresses and vulnerabilities of late life make them more exaggerated and apparent. This was the case with Sally.

Aunt Sally was known as the shy one in the Bond family. Retiring and modest, she had remained unmarried, living with a domineering younger sister who took care of all their outside chores. The sister was the only person whom Sally felt safe going out with, and in their thirty-some years together she never left the house with anyone else.

In her sixties, the sister married a widower and moved into a retirement community, leaving Sally alone for the first time. Although she was in good health and mentally competent, she quickly began displaying signs of agoraphobia. Her niece brought her to see me after she discovered that Sally was eating spoiled food that had been left in the house since her sister's departure, because she was too shy to go out in public to shop or ask for assistance.

At their visit, the niece had to speak for Sally, a tiny woman with a fine-boned face and trembling hands. She could not look me in the eye or directly answer any of my questions, except to acknowledge that she had always suffered anxiety about leaving her living quarters and considered herself safe only when she was in the confines of her room. At one point during our talk, she said she was dizzy and asked if she could leave.

In cases such as Sally's, symptoms may be masked or covered by spouses and family members until they are revealed in the isolation of late life. Sally had been shielded from her disorder for years by her sister; she would have eaten rotten food before leaving her house and asking for help.

## Social Phobias

These are often characterized by a potent, ongoing fear of strangers, unfamiliar social situations, or speaking or performing in public. People with these syndromes may have anxiety about voicing their opinions, using public bathrooms, or eating in front of others, because of a fear of being judged, embarrassed, humiliated, or evaluated. Sufferers feel that they are on display whenever they are required to be involved in group interaction or small talk and may develop severe anxiety symptoms if forced into such situations. In the elderly, social phobias about activities such as eating or speaking can be accentuated by dentures or other physical disabilities.

Social phobias do not arise from poor social skills; rather, it's the chronic anxiety about these skills—whether a person will appear foolish or be judged—that characterizes the disorder and makes a parent avoidant and withdrawn.

In younger years, individuals with this type of phobia may be viewed as shy and introverted types who don't put themselves forward for notice, attention, or promotion. After retirement, phobia sufferers may avoid people entirely or limit their social contacts to family.

This was the case with Eric, a businessman whose success had been curtailed by his severe phobia of speaking in public. Throughout his career he'd forfeited advances and promotions rather than take on responsibility that involved appearing in front of any type of audience, no matter how small. He'd enrolled in Dale Carnegie courses and Toastmasters, and watched while his colleagues succeeded and moved on. But his problem was more severe than simple stage fright, and could not be solved by preparation and practice. Whenever he tried to talk in front of others, his hands trembled and his heart beat so rapidly, he admitted, that "all I wanted to do was run."

His phobia impaired his ability to rise in his company, where he remained at a junior-level position for thirty years. To his embarrassment, his wife had to work several jobs in order for the family to make ends meet.

After he retired in his late sixties, Eric suffered a massive coronary, and his social anxiety grew markedly worse. His daughter reported: "He won't even go out to eat with us anymore. He doesn't like anyone to look at him, so he stopped going to church, too."

Always a social drinker, Eric began mixing prescription drugs with his nightly scotch. His daughter decided it was time to bring him in for treatment when she found him so overmedicated one morning that she could barely wake him.

# WHAT CAUSES PHOBIAS?

## GENES AND PHOBIA

Genetics is assumed to play a role in the development of phobias; having a close relative—mother, father, sister, brother—with social phobia, for example, increases the risk of phobia development.[2]

Research by Harvard's Dr. Jerome Kagan has also shown that sociability and shyness are temperamental traits that are enduring and have a biological basis. In response to new situations, shy children exhibit a higher heart rate and a more rapid increase in pulse, as opposed to outgoing children. This overactive stress response may predispose a person to develop anxiety disorders such as phobias later in life.[3]

## EARLY LIFE EXPERIENCES

In combination with biological factors, studies show that phobias may have a correlation to environmental stresses such as early parental loss or family violence.[4] Agoraphobia in particular, which compels sufferers to stay near a "safe" haven, is theorized to stem from early-childhood insecurities caused by neglect, abuse, or abandonment. But agoraphobia may develop at any time in adulthood, even old age, if a severe threat causes a person to become anxious when they leave the confines of their home.

### NEUROBIOLOGY

Brain chemistry can make a person genetically susceptible to exaggerated anxiety reactions that contribute to phobias. Irregularities in the levels of the brain neurotransmitters serotonin, dopamine, and GABA are believed to be particularly implicated in phobias. Research has also shown that social-disorder sufferers exhibit greater activation in a part of the brain called the amygdala in response to harsh versus accepting or happy facial expressions.[5]

### TRAUMA

Phobias can be caused by observed or experienced traumatic events, such as accidents or sudden illnesses. In a simple phobia, a painful past incident is sometimes the clear cause. The frightening experience of being in a car crash, for example, develops into an association with automobiles and fear. The avoidance of cars distances the person from the anxiety-producing situation, so that when he is next "exposed" to a car and the anxiety returns, the avoidance is reinforced.

Studies suggest that traumatic events leave an imprint on the brain and that these memories may later trigger phobias. Fear of stimuli previously considered innocent is believed to be a result of experience-induced changes in brain synapses.[6]

## TREATMENT

Research suggests that a combination of psychotherapy and pharmacotherapy is more effective in treating phobic disorders than either on its own.

## Psychotherapeutic Techniques

### *Best Bets*

**Cognitive-behavior techniques** are the treatment of choice for phobia sufferers, focusing on changing both thinking patterns *and* actions. This type of therapy shows a patient how to confront and eventually overcome his fears.

Sufferers of specific phobias often cope by avoiding a feared situation or object. But this is a way of perpetuating phobias, not curing them. **Exposure therapy** is a method that can teach people to overcome phobias for good.

In fact, some experts claim that they can treat a severe phobia in a matter of days using CBT and actually taking a height-phobic person to a high place, for example. By repeatedly surviving these experiences, a patient eventually forms new memories to replace the terrifying, phobic ones. This technique, where a patient is directly exposed to a feared situation or object all at once, is called **flooding.**

In other cases, a patient is confronted with a feared object or situation, gradually or through imagery, composing a "hierarchy" of steps toward the feared object or situation, beginning with the least and advancing to the most feared.

In Sally's case this involved imaginary exposure to the outside world she so feared. She was asked to break down her feared activity—leaving her house and walking to the mailbox on the corner—into the following small, incremental steps, each of which she would repeat five times before moving on to the next one:

■ Standing outside her front door for a minute.
■ Standing on her front porch for a minute.
■ Standing on the first step for a minute.
■ Walking down the steps and standing at the bottom for a minute.
■ Walking to the curb and standing there for a minute.
■ Walking down the sidewalk to the next house, standing for a minute.

- Walking two houses down, standing for a minute.
- Walking to the corner to the mailbox.

First, Sally went through each of these steps in her mind until she could visualize herself completing them without anxiety.

The next component involved real-life exposure: she completed each step five times, first with a trusted friend or family member, then on her own.

She didn't advance to the next step until she felt perfectly comfortable with the previous one. She visualized a relaxing scene that she could retreat to—a peaceful mountaintop—whenever she experienced any anxiety symptoms.

In the cognitive component of CBT, a parent is taught how to reduce anxiety, minimize negative thinking, and reframe a problem. In phobic disorders, sufferers tend to develop false, exaggerated, and destructive ways of thinking about a problem. A phobic mother might think: "I can't ever visit my daughter again because I'm terrified of taking the elevator up to her apartment." A social-phobia sufferer makes such statements as "If I go out in public, I'll look ridiculous and make a fool of myself."

My patient Sally was taught how to recognize such anxiety-provoking thoughts as "If I go out to the park, I'll be overwhelmed by the crowds there" and reframe them with the positive replacement: "If I go to the park, I'll see my friend and get fresh air, both of which will make me feel healthy and happier."

These reframings, combined with relaxation techniques such as deep abdominal breathing and positive visualizations, eventually led to the behavior component of her therapy.

## Pharmacological Treatments

Medications can help alleviate anxiety symptoms and allow a parent to confront phobic situations. They can provide temporary control over a phobia, but they will not cure it.

## *Best Bets*

**SSRIs** are my first choice when I'm dealing with the anxiety symptoms associated with phobias. SSRIs help restore the balance of serotonin, which can reduce the symptoms of anxiety and depression. They do not produce the withdrawal problems of the benzodiazepines nor the cardiac side effects of the tricyclics. SSRIs are also effective in treating the depression and anxiety that are often features of the disorder.

Paxil is an SSRI specifically approved for social phobias, as is Effexor, a newer dual-agent drug, which boosts both norepinephrine and serotonin and is therefore known as an SSNRI.

Other SSRIs have also been shown to be effective, including Zoloft, Prozac, Celexa, and Luvox. Side effects may include nausea, insomnia, headache, and loss of sexual desire.

A parent should be reminded that it may take up to eight weeks to experience the full effects of these drugs. If one SSRI doesn't work, another should be tried. Sally found relief from her lifetime phobias with Paxil XR, an extended relief version of the older drug.

### BETA-BLOCKERS (INDERAL — PROPRANOLOL)

**Inderal** is the drug of choice for people who fear specific social circumstances, such as giving a speech or attending a social gathering. Inderal relieves such stage-fright symptoms as blushing, stuttering, and racing heart. These drugs reduce the adrenaline rush and hyperarousal symptoms that are a feature of performance phobias. They are fast-acting and nonaddictive, but caution must be used with those who have other health conditions, such as cardiac problems, asthma, or vascular disease.

## *Other Choices*

**Benzodiazepines** such as Xanax and Valium, both approved for treating anxiety disorders, were once the mainstay of phobia treatment, since they can reduce situation-specific social phobia within minutes. They are fast-acting and effective for eradicating the fear and anxiety related to phobic behavior.

However, these drugs should only be used in short-term situations with the elderly, since daily use can lead to physical dependence. They also have troublesome side effects in late life—such as falling, memory problems, and confusion.

Withdrawal symptoms may occur when a patient abruptly discontinues taking these antianxiety medications. Mild symptoms of withdrawal include rebound anxiety, involuntary movements, insomnia, restlessness, and perceptual changes. Severe symptoms can include confusion and seizures.

**MAOIs.** Some experts consider Nardil, an MAOI that boosts all three neurotransmitters, the drug of choice for phobia disorder, particularly social anxiety. My concern, however, is with the cumbersome dietary restrictions that are necessary in order to safely take this drug. MAOIs require a restricted diet that rules out wine, cheese, and beer, which contain tyramine, a substance that may cause a dangerous increase in blood pressure.

# PROBLEMS THAT CAN MIMIC
# OR COEXIST WITH PHOBIAS

**Depression and other anxiety disorders.** Phobic sufferers who undergo years of disabling fear and anxiety are also likely to suffer from depression, which may require separate treatment. Those with social phobia also have a high risk for suffering from other psychiatric conditions, including panic disorder, agoraphobia, obsessive-compulsive disorder, and general anxiety disorder.

**Adjustment anxiety** is a common, transient anxiety that occurs when a patient moves, loses a spouse, or becomes ill. This anxiety is situational and passes in a short time without treatment or medication.

**Substance abuse and alcohol abuse.** Over-the-counter medication and alcohol may be used by a parent to mask the fearfulness and terror of phobias.

Social phobia may be mistakenly diagnosed as excessive shyness. But simple shyness does not present the physical symptoms that are a common feature of social phobia, including trembling, sweating, and heart palpitations.

**Attention deficit disorder** often coexists with phobias.

**Parkinson's disease,** which is linked with low dopamine levels, has been found to often coexist with social phobia.

---

### Questions to Ask Your Parent
### If You Suspect Phobia Disorder

▪ Is there a specific situation or object that you feel severe dread about—such as getting in an elevator or seeing a spider?

▪ Are you finding it more difficult to leave the house because of feelings of fear?

▪ Do you feel an overwhelming shyness about eating, speaking, or appearing in public?

▪ Do you have strong fears that you realize intellectually are unreasonable and foolish but that you still can't resist?

▪ Are you finding your day-to-day functioning hampered by a persistent fear or dread?

▪ Have you missed out on an enjoyable activity lately because of an unreasonable terror?

▪ Do you spend a portion of time each day preoccupied with a dreaded situation or object and ways to avoid it?

---

## HOW YOU CAN HELP

**Initiate treatment.** Given the socially avoidant and fearful nature of these disorders, a parent may be extremely reluctant to seek help, and you may need to be the one to initiate treatment. Calling clinicians to make appointments, accompanying a parent, and helping him talk to the clinician can all be especially beneficial.

**Monitor treatment.** An agoraphobic mother may not even want to leave the house to fill prescriptions or attend therapy. Helping a parent care for these basic necessities may require hiring a home health aide, a driver, or enlisting a prescription-delivery service.

**Act as a support person.** Offer to accompany your parent when embarking on an exposure venture or an event that she feels particularly anxious about attending.

**Be positive and praise treatment efforts.** Since failure to comply with treatment is common among the elderly, encourage consistency of medication or cognitive-behavior therapy. Let a parent know that the treatment prognosis is good for phobias, especially if the patient is determined to work hard.

**Be on the lookout for substance abuse.** The fearful nature of these disorders may drive parents to overmedicate or mix alcohol and drugs. Keep an eye out for weight or behavior changes.

### SYMPTOMS OF PHOBIA DISORDER

| PHYSIOLOGICAL | BEHAVIORAL | COGNITIVE |
|---|---|---|
| Trembling | Avoids phobic trigger | Persistent, unreasonable fear and dread |
| Sweating | | |
| | Self-isolates | Fear is recognized as unreasonable |
| Stammer | | |
| Rapid heartbeat | | |

# PART
# THREE

■ ■ ■

# 10

# PSYCHOTHERAPEUTIC INTERVENTIONS

I'm often surprised at how rarely anxious seniors and their families consider psychotherapeutic options. A daughter of one of my patients laughed at the notion that her anxious eighty-year-old mother might benefit from psychotherapy.

"I'm the one in therapy because of *her,*" she said.

Her mother concurred with her. "I'm an old dog; at this point, I'm not going to change my tricks."

The notion that the elderly are rigid, unchangeable, and unable to alter behaviors and thought patterns they've possessed for many years is not uncommon. Freud himself believed a person couldn't benefit from psychotherapy after forty, since too many events had already occurred in his life.

However, research shows that older people are actually more likely to finish a course of counseling, and that the rates for recovery in both older and younger people are about the same.

Indeed, there are a number of reasons why these interventions are a good first resort for seniors with mild anxiety or depression.

Chief among them is that many of these treatments can be incorporated into a parent's long-term self-care. If a parent learns new techniques to cope with anxiety-inducing behavior or thought patterns, this learning can be long-lasting, even permanent.

Cognitive-behavior techniques such as thought-stopping or gradual exposure can develop into lifelong coping tools, to be used whenever a patient needs them. And if talk or group therapy is found effective in dealing with a patient's isolated, withdrawn behavior or generalized anxiety, it can be utilized for ongoing support and treatment in a community setting. This is opposed to the benefits of most medications, which disappear once they're stopped.

Unlike drugs, psychotherapeutic interventions also have few adverse side effects, especially when performed by an experienced counselor. Additionally, they're beneficial for patients who can't take medication because of interactions with other drugs or preexisting illnesses. Some patients are also strongly opposed to any type of psychiatric medication for religious reasons.

Finally, just as understanding the biological basis of syndromes can be helpful in understanding an anxious parent, so can being aware of the psychological issues at the root of certain disorders. Discovering the trauma underlying her mother's PTSD, and learning what steps she could take to master the situation, allowed Lili to be a more empathic and sympathetic daughter.

"My mother's fearfulness always drove me crazy when I was growing up. I thought she was trying to get attention. When a doctor diagnosed her as having posttraumatic stress, I couldn't believe it. 'What's been so traumatic in her life?' I asked. I was floored when my father told me that she'd been sexually abused by an uncle when she was young. This changed my whole view of my mother. I don't react like I used to when she has one of her spells. I can see how this has scarred her."

For some families, accepting that a parent needs therapy requires a readjustment of their point of view: they have to view the parent not just as a satellite around their personal orbit, but as an autonomous adult with long-term issues and problems that often predate them.

On the other hand, there are also several drawbacks to psychotherapeutic techniques. They often take longer than medication to be effective, and may require both an ongoing commitment and frequent office visits.

Additionally, some parents find any type of psychological treatment too threatening and feel uncomfortable divulging personal information to a therapist or doctor. In the past, some therapists induced more problems than they helped because they only focused on uncovering problems and didn't offer strategies for learning new, more adaptive approaches. With more focused, goal-oriented therapies, this has become less problematic, especially with clinicians who have specific experience in treating older individuals.

## COGNITIVE-BEHAVIOR THERAPY

Experts were once divided into two camps regarding the most effective way of treating anxiety disorders. One side believed that having insight into the patient's problem and learning to think about it differently was the most important element. The other camp insisted that it was more important to change behavior, and that thinking patterns and moods would alter in response.

It now appears that both sides were right; if you help people change *both* their thinking and the way they act, the combination is more effective and long-lasting than either component alone. Many therapists utilize this combined method, cognitive-behavior therapy (CBT), to treat anxiety disorders.

Cognitive-behavior therapy proves that people have the power to change their thinking and control how they respond to stress. Studies show that these techniques, which focus on concrete behavior and thought, are as helpful as medication in treating such conditions as mild anxiety and depression. Furthermore, if these therapies are combined with medication when the symptoms are more severe, the treatment is better than either counseling or medication alone.

Blanche was a divorced woman of sixty-six, whose life had been severely curtailed by serious agoraphobia and generalized anxiety disorder (GAD). She had always been fretful about her health—her children considered her a hypochondriac—but her symptoms worsened after her divorce, cascading from a chronic gastritis that she was sure was a sign of cancer to a shifting set of aches and pains that could never be specifically diagnosed. By the time she was in her sixties, she'd worked out an elaborate system so that she could essentially remain isolated inside her house: her family visited her monthly, and she had her food and medications delivered. The only event she regularly left her apartment for was a weekly session with a psychoanalyst she'd been seeing for twenty years.

This limited, isolated existence had started to become untenable. Her health had begun deteriorating in earnest, but she couldn't be convinced to see a specialist other than her therapist. When her daughter finally managed to bring her to me, I found a pale woman with dark rings under her eyes.

"She's been in talk therapy for years," her daughter reported. "By now, we understand her dreams and fears and where they come from. We've found out that her rigid mother made her childhood miserable and that her divorce was traumatic. We understand all this, but she's still stuck inside the house, a worry machine."

The fact is that many anxiety syndromes are tenacious disorders that can't be solved simply by plumbing the past or providing empathy. Blanche needed much more specific and directed treatment.

It was not until she began attending a cognitive-behavior program geared to her unique problems that she began to make substantial improvement.

## THE C IN CBT

The C in CBT stands for "cognitive"; this is the component of therapy that focuses on how your parent thinks. Anxious parents have learned or been taught maladaptive thought patterns that cause or contribute to their being fearful or depressed. They often emphasize emotions over thought, and are unable to act in a clear-headed fashion once they become upset. Their feelings, in effect, carry them away, resulting in panic, phobias, and other anxiety symptoms. Cognitive techniques focus on teaching them to evaluate these runaway feelings, irrational fears, and negative thoughts and finding new ways of dealing with them.

Anxious patients are often flooded with powerful, negative thoughts that feed on one another, spiraling into a state of confusion, distress, and emotional paralysis. The patient who has sustained himself for years on an internal diet of such inner messages as "I'm a loser," "I'm damaged," "This is too much for me" has become enmeshed in a self-perpetuating cycle of anxiety. Severing these negative loops requires the kind of focused approach cognitive therapy provides.

With these techniques, patients are taught to identify patterns of thinking that are ultimately harmful. They may be instructed to keep a journal of their thoughts and to question the negative assumptions that underlie them.

Once this takes place, they can be taught new, more effective strategies for thinking about problems and ultimately replace the negative, self-destructive thought patterns with methods of positive coping.

In effect, the therapist is teaching a patient to discard the following types of distressing, anxiety-provoking thought patterns and profiles and to replace them with alternative approaches that are more effective.

# ANXIETY-PROVOKING PATTERNS AND PROFILES

## THE OVERWORRIER: WHAT IF?

Catastrophic, "what if" thinking is a feature of many anxiety disorders, particularly GAD and panic. Overworried parents chronically exaggerate the odds of negative outcomes at the same time as they minimize their ability to handle them. They don't do this because they *want* to, but because this is how they have learned to think.

A common thought sequence that produces anxiety in a parent with GAD might be "My head hurts. What if I'm dying of brain cancer? I'll go to pieces and won't be able to handle it."

Cognitive techniques counter these thoughts by breaking them down and examining their validity. For example:

*In your past life, how often have headaches indicated that you have cancer?* (Answer: "I've often had headaches in the past, and they've never been caused by cancer.")

*What are the odds that the headache is due to something else, such as seasonal allergy or stress?* (Answer: "Since it's spring, and I'm allergic to pollen, there's a good chance my headaches are caused by allergies.")

*In the unlikely event that a headache did equal cancer, what could you do about it?* (Answer: "Since many cancers are curable, I'd most likely enter into a partnership with my doctor and family and receive treatment.")

Catastrophic thinking in people with OCD can cause exaggerated feelings of responsibility. One woman believed that if she didn't continually call to remind her husband to wear his seat belt he would be involved in a fatal accident. Working with a therapist and learning ways to counteract destructive thinking allowed her to break these patterns.

Similarly, a patient suffering from panic attacks often misinterprets bodily symptoms as indications of an oncoming attack. Cognitive therapy aims to eliminate these misinterpretations and break the cycle of increased anxiety that occurs in anticipation of these events.

When a panicked patient says, "My heart's beating fast, I can't breathe, I'm going to die!" her panicked thoughts lead to the release of stress hormones that further accelerates her symptoms.

By replacing such panicked thoughts with positive coping statements, such as "This is only panic; my body's feeling the effects of adrenaline. If I practice deep breathing and other relaxation techniques, I can ward off this attack," she is actually able to lessen the physiological response to the worry and avoid the physical symptoms (rapid heartbeat, accelerated breathing) that signal a full-blown attack.

A socially phobic patient might say, "I can't go to the retirement party. What if I make a fool of myself and start to sweat and tremble? Everybody will judge me!"

Cognitive coping statements to replace these negative thoughts could be: "If I look like a fool it won't kill me. I can handle feeling uncomfortable for a while. And even if I do get nervous, I can go to another room and practice my relaxation exercises."

## THE VICTIM: I CAN'T

The mantra of victimized thought is "I can't." Depressed patients often engage in this kind of thinking and use absolutes such as "never," "nothing," "always": "I'm *never* a success at anything." "People are *always* criticizing me." "*Nothing* ever improves in my life."

Parents who use victimized thought focus only on negative aspects of themselves, in a process called **filtering.** Showing why such thoughts aren't true—and helping a parent change them—is one of the main goals of cognitive therapy.

A therapist counters victimized thinking with concrete, real-life examples:

*"I'm never a success at anything":* You've been involved in a stable marriage for forty-five years and raised two successful children.

*"People are always criticizing me":* In the last year, you've only been overtly criticized once, by your sister.

*"Nothing ever improves":* You recently received a promotion at your job.

The goal in counteracting filtering isn't to convince the anxious person that he's never failed or made mistakes, but rather to teach him to have a more balanced assessment of his strengths and limitations.

## THE JUDGER: I SHOULD

The judger is a perfectionist who turns scrutiny onto herself and creates more anxiety and fear. Her negative self-evaluations ignore positive attributes and create anxiety by focusing on flaws and limitations.

The judger says: "I have no excuse for being tense. I should be calm instead of fearful. I should be able to handle this."

Cognitive techniques focus on affirmative coping statements, such as "I'm all right as I am. I do the best I can. Even if I do become anxious, I still do a good job. In fact, sometimes I do better when I'm a little nervous."

The goal of the therapist is to help the patient realize how negative ways of thinking both cause and maintain anxiety and depression, and to show that these negative thought patterns can be consciously changed with practice.

## THE CONCLUSION-JUMPER

The overgeneralizer, or conclusion-jumper, is another expert at quickly accelerating anxiety and panic. He says: "I had a panic attack the last time I drove over the bridge, and now it's going to happen every time."

This kind of thinking can be countered by rational questioning: "What's the evidence that one panic attack on a bridge means a lifetime of them? Haven't you driven over many bridges in your life without having panic attacks?"

It usually works to replace these overgeneralized thoughts with positive coping statements. Instead of simply stating, "I'm not going to panic when I cross the bridge," the statement should be framed in a positive way: "I will be calm and serene as I cross the bridge."

In the cognitive technique called **reframing,** a therapist listens to a patient's irrational or negative beliefs and fears and tries to conceptualize the situation in a more positive way.

An agoraphobic mother says: "I don't want to eat out because the restaurant will be so crowded that it's going to make me nervous." A cognitive therapist would help her turn her thoughts around and focus on the positive aspects of the outing, so that she might say: "I'll be able to visit with my friends at the restaurant and enjoy food I can't make for myself at home."

A behavioral component would be for her to schedule the dinner an hour earlier, when the restaurant isn't so crowded, or to be accompanied by a support person who can drive her home if she becomes panicked.

A person suffering from performance anxiety who says, "I feel so nervous before I speak in public that I'm sure I'll make a fool of myself," is taught to reframe his reaction into: "A little anxiety improves my performance." The added behavioral techniques of progressive relaxation and slow abdominal breathing can help the person control any uncomfortable anxiety.

**Thought-stopping** is a cognitive technique for suppressing or switching off the cascading flow of anxiety-provoking thoughts. It involves disrupting negative thoughts by saying, either out loud or to oneself, "No! Stop!" whenever an anxious thought pattern emerges. Another method is to snap a rubber band worn around the wrist whenever anxious thoughts arise.

Used with a PTSD father, for example, thought-stopping should occur as soon as he finds his thoughts returning to the horrifying car accident that once traumatized him. When he finds himself reliving the incident or his thoughts begin to wander back to the highway, he is told to snap the rubber band and tell himself firmly, "Stop it! No!"

## BEHAVIORAL TECHNIQUES

**Behavioral therapy** focuses on altering feelings by first changing behaviors, often by bringing a patient gradually into contact with a feared object or situation. Facing down these demons is often the ultimate cure for fears and phobias and can be a liberating act for a fearful older parent. This approach contrasts with therapies that first focus on expressing or understanding a parent's emotional response or on uncovering the psychological causes of symptoms. In my experience, behavioral techniques are especially helpful for treating individuals with phobias and those who tend to focus too much on their emotions.

**Exposure therapy** involves therapeutically confronting a feared object, situation, or past trauma by either imagining it in great detail or visiting locales that are strong reminders of the experience. By taking small, incremental steps toward the feared object or situation, a patient is able to face, and ultimately gain control of, his fear.

If your father has a shark phobia, for example, a good therapist wouldn't simply push him into the Atlantic and wish him luck. She'd start by talking to him in her office about sharks, showing him an informative book about sharks, telling him about a shark's life cycle, the way it cares for its young, where it swims and feeds. Next, she might show him a nature documentary that features sharks; perhaps she'd accompany him to a natural history museum where he could see a model of one. Finally, she might take him to an aquarium where he could see a live shark swim in front of him. At this point, your father may not be ready to dive into the ocean to swim with these creatures, but he would have been desensitized to his intense fear of them. It would now be more *under his control.*

Experts call these steps toward reaching a feared goal or object a **hierarchy.** Nancy, a phobic mother, used exposure to reach her goal—taking an airplane flight from Kansas City to Omaha to see her granddaughter graduate. Her task was broken down into a series of eight to twelve graduated steps, starting with the simplest and ending with the most anxiety-provoking . . . her goal. A trusted support person or partner, in this case her sister, accompanied her during this process.

For her plane phobia, these steps were to:

- Watch a documentary or instructional video of a plane taking off and landing
- Drive by the airport with a support person and watch planes taking off and landing
- Park in the airport lot with a support partner and watch planes taking off and landing
- Go inside the airport and stay for ten minutes
- Enter a plane on the ground with a support partner and sit in a seat for ten minutes
- Enter a grounded plane without a support partner and sit in a seat for fifteen minutes
- Take a short flight of less than thirty minutes with a support partner
- Take a longer flight with a support partner
- Take a flight alone

In **imaginary exposure,** a patient is subjected to the feared situation or object in his mind through imagination.

A therapist asks a parent to visualize the situation or object that produces anxiety, then teaches him relaxation techniques to handle his feelings. The goal is to lessen the anxiety a parent feels when faced with a feared situation or object—to gradually *desensitize* him to its power.

For a phobia that is difficult to confront in a gradual way, a therapist might have a patient use imaginary exposure, linked with steps that he would eventually take in real life. For example, another patient of mine had a phobia of overseas flights, but wanted to take one in order to visit her son who had moved to Rome.

The following steps could be used:

- Relax completely, take deep abdominal breaths.
- Visualize that you are walking on a beautiful, relaxing beach at sunset—the ocean is lapping beside you, a cool breeze is in your hair. You are completely calm and at peace.
- See an image of a plane in front of you. You are looking at it through a glass window. See yourself watching it as calmly as possible; if you feel no anxiety, advance to the next step.
- If you *do* feel anxiety, try to remain in the fearful scene a few more moments, breathing in and relaxing. Use positive coping statements such as "I am relaxing," "I am calm." Then retreat to your peaceful beach scene. Go back and forth between the fearful scene and your peaceful scene until you are totally relaxed. Then proceed to the next step on your hierarchy ladder.
- See yourself driving to the airport, parking, and walking into the terminal.
- See yourself walking onto a grounded plane and sitting in the seat.
- Imagine yourself seated in a plane, being buckled in, and the flight attendant shutting the door.
- See yourself in a plane that takes off and flies for a short period, then returns safely and lands.
- Finally, visualize yourself taking off on a long flight and landing safely.

The opposite of imaginary exposure, **flooding** is a technique in which a patient is exposed directly—and all at once—to a feared stimuli. Boston University's Dr. David Barlow promotes a type of flooding that he refers to as "talking to the amygdala" to cure severe phobias. Based on the theory that avoiding what you fear is not only futile but doesn't cure phobias or fears, Barlow would take a patient suffering from a height phobia directly to a high spot and let him see how it feels to survive it, rather than simply reassuring him that such a place is safe. After repeatedly surviving these experiences, a patient eventually forms new memories to replace the terrifying old ones.[1]

In another, related method, pills and games are used to help conquer fear. A reality game that simulates an agoraphobic's worst nightmare—riding a glass elevator inside the courtyard of a high-rise hotel—is combined with a drug that reportedly revs up certain learning circuits in the brain. Researchers gave a drug called DCS to subjects terrified of heights, before having them don virtual-reality goggles and taking them up in elevators as far as they could go. While subjects who took the drug didn't find their anxiety reduced in the same way as they did with Valium or other related drugs, they became progressively bolder in subsequent virtual sessions. And, even more important, they were twice as likely to make strides in real-life situations. Those who took DCS were twice as likely to use an elevator or drive on high bridges in the real world.[2]

Exposure is based on the notion that anxiety is reduced after there is sufficient contact with a feared object. A parent suffering from OCD who is terrified of germy objects such as money is required to remain in contact with it until the anxiety is eventually lessened.

To work best, exposure is often combined with **response prevention,** in which a ritualistic behavior is blocked. In the case of a mother suffering from OCD who's terrified of money, she would be required not only to handle dollar bills (perhaps after a gradual exposure that involved first looking at pictures of money, then looking at but not touching money, then holding the bills in her hand), but would also be blocked from the ritualized washing that had previously followed such contact. As I note in the chapter on OCD, these approaches are not helpful for everyone, but some individuals are able to become much more functional after such therapy.

**Habit reversal** is a behavioral method that can help a patient eradicate anxiety-related rituals and habits. For a panic disorder, a patient would be asked to call a friend instead of the emergency room whenever he feels an attack coming on, or to take a brisk walk instead of freezing up and counting his pulse. In OCD, habit reversal might involve the replacement of ritual with a similar, non-OCD behavior, such as rubbing hand lotion into hands instead of compulsively washing them with soap and water.

**Contingency management** is based on the tenet that a rewarded behavior is more likely to occur. In cases of social phobia, a parent might be rewarded $5 each time he manages to leave the house to attend a group meeting and required to pay that much whenever he succumbs to anxiety and remains home instead.

Incorporating costs and rewards in ritual prevention might involve a parent suffering from OCD paying his spouse every time he engages in ritualized checking and being taken out to dinner every day that he does not engage in compulsive behavior.

## PSYCHOTHERAPY

Psychotherapy, talk therapy, and interpersonal therapy all refer to a type of therapeutic approach in which the primary active ingredient is a relationship rooted in discussion between a therapist and patient.

Psychotherapy utilizes techniques that are designed to alter emotions, thoughts, and habits. It builds on the idea that if one knows the source of a problem, it's much easier to address and change it. Psychotherapy can relieve symptoms of emotional distress and increase self-understanding and promote emotional growth. Encouragement, support, empathic listening, reassurance, and guidance are among the benefits psychotherapy can provide for the isolated elderly.

Psychotherapy can benefit fretful, lonely seniors who need to talk out their feelings about family, illness, or financial concerns with a nonjudgmental listener.

"I have so many worries that no one knows about—not even my kids," Ann, one patient, told me. "Sometimes I just need to get things off my chest without being concerned about how someone else will react. Every time I have a visit with my therapist, I feel better."

Short-term, insight-oriented therapy can be especially helpful for seniors. Often an **acute crisis intervention** or brief encounter of one or two talk-therapy sessions by a trained geriatric therapist can alleviate certain anxiety symptoms right away.

A patient of mine, Nilda, who was traumatized after a hit-and-run accident, was able to benefit from half a dozen of these sessions. She was able to talk about how vulnerable she'd felt since the accident and consider ways to prevent herself from becoming permanently trapped by these feelings. "If I hadn't talked about my accident right away, I think I might have become paralyzed by fear. Because I faced the emotions that were coming out in me in therapy, I didn't have the chance to brood and isolate myself."

A contrasting approach is provided by **problem-solving therapy,** which helps people focus on and solve current problems. This therapy is based on the assumption that reviewing the past has little or no benefit in addressing current problems and helping people change. This therapy identifies the difficulties people are currently experiencing, the elements in their lives that are contributing to them, and then focuses on what aspects of their lives can be changed.

One patient, Pat, who found herself anxious and lonely since her move to an assisted-living facility, was helped when her therapist came up with several very specific steps that she could immediately take to help her broaden her social sphere, such as: calling the recreation center for a schedule of events, inviting a next-door neighbor over for coffee; and joining a volunteer phone tree that checks on homebound seniors.

The focus of this therapy is on concrete suggestions, not the negative or anxious way a patient is thinking.

In follow-up sessions, Pat and her therapist would determine whether she had taken the steps they agreed upon, and, if not, what barriers were preventing it. They might either come up with a new list of steps or keep the same list and monitor over the ensuing weeks whether progress was being made.

**Psychoanalytic therapy** is a particular type of counseling, originated by

Freud, that focuses on the belief that early life experiences are important in understanding current emotions, and that unresolved conflicts from childhood lead to depression or anxiety in later life.

A psychoanalytic approach views the development of a disorder such as GAD as related to conflicts that are unresolved and unconscious, such as an event early in a patient's life that continues to be upsetting. This could be a developmental lapse, such as separation from a loved one or object, as was the case with Marie, who lost her widowed mother when she was a toddler and was subsequently raised in an orphanage. Older than the other children, she was never chosen for adoption and grew up anxious and fretful, never feeling she had enough support or love.

Even though she married later in life and had a large family, her anxiety never left her, and by her seventies, widowed and living alone, she suffered from a serious case of generalized anxiety.

In supportive counseling, Marie discovered that she had not only felt abandoned all those years, but had also harbored the worry that she had perhaps been responsible for the death of her mother. Once she was able to explore these issues in treatment, she could face her unexpressed grief and recognize that there was no basis for her feelings of responsibility.

Psychoanalytic therapy is usually a long-term commitment, and it is generally less effective in treating late-life anxiety disorders than cognitive-behavior therapy. While it can be helpful to understand how a phobia is rooted in childhood, this is usually not as effective as facing the feared situation directly.

However, some patients find that they enjoy the chance to review their lives and to gain an understanding of their current feelings and behaviors based on the insights they gain in this kind of treatment.

**Group treatment** is commonly used in veteran and crisis clinics for assault and abuse victims, as well as in support groups for diseases like Alzheimer's and cancer. Under the leadership of a therapist, a group of peers (often six to ten people) meets regularly to provide a therapeutic setting in which participants share problems and symptoms with others who have undergone the same experiences.

The benefits of group therapy are the support that comes from knowing that peers are having similar problems ("I'm not the only one who . . ."), the solutions suggested by other group's members, and, occasionally, being confronted by peers when a person is either not trying to change or is acting in a way that is destructive or undermining his progress.

By providing increased support and social interaction, this type of treatment can be especially helpful for isolated seniors. Realizing that others share their symptoms can be cathartic for a patient such as Keith, whose phobias had made him so fearful that he often didn't leave his apartment for weeks on end. Weekly group therapy at a local senior center opened up a new world for him. "I couldn't believe there were so many other people who felt as trapped as I did. I don't feel so odd anymore. I made friends, and I got out of the house every Tuesday morning."

In my experience, however, group therapy isn't always the best choice with certain disorders, especially for seniors suffering from PTSD, because it sometimes *encourages* sufferers to revisit and ruminate about their traumas.

This happened with my patient Rich, who found in his veterans' group an all-too-sympathetic venue when it came to rehashing and refocusing on traumatic events during the Korean War that had precipitated his PTSD symptoms in the first place. Instead of helping him, these weekly meetings had the effect of preoccupying him even further with the past. It wasn't until he became actively involved in a behavioral regimen, where his maladaptive behaviors were weakened and eventually eliminated, that he found lasting relief. Groups that encourage people to change the way they're thinking and behaving are more helpful in this circumstance.

## SPECIAL ISSUES OF LATE LIFE

The use of psychotherapy can bring up special issues for seniors. Revealing emotional problems can be an uncomfortable experience for some parents, who see a stigma attached to mental health problems, or worry that they have Alzheimer's or are developing dementia. A parent may be more likely to confide in a trusted primary-care doctor, who can then make the psychological referral. Family involvement can also increase the effectiveness of psychotherapy.

Some psychotherapeutic treatments may need to be delivered at a slower pace with the anxious elderly. Consideration may also need to be given to practical issues such as poor vision, fear of travel and crowds, and anxiety about working with new clinicians.

## A Cognitive-Behavior Exercise, Combining Reframing, Visualization, and Contingency Management Techniques for a Mother's PTSD

Ever since Cassie had her purse snatched while walking down a local street, she's been terrified of leaving the house or driving, and finds herself repeatedly replaying the scene in her mind. She's curtailed many of her everyday activities, such as grocery shopping and visiting friends, and has become increasingly isolated.

The following is a cognitive-behavior **reframing** technique that helped her anxiety symptoms:

- Identify the cognitions or thoughts that you have when you think about going out ("I'll be knocked down again"; "I'll break my hip"; "I'll lose all my money"; "I'll be killed this time").
- Identify the negative aspects of these thoughts and examine their reality. For example, the likelihood of being mugged again is low, especially if steps are taken to be safe—for example, by going out only in the morning and being accompanied by a friend.
- Break down the activity of leaving the house into small steps (i.e., walking out the door, standing on the porch, going down the steps, walking thirty feet down the sidewalk).
- Learn a relaxation technique, such as: Visualize yourself walking down the street feeling as confident and relaxed as if you were strolling on the most beautiful ocean beach, surrounded by good friends and family. When you think about going out, do the relaxation exercise. Later, when you take the first step out of the house, you should again do the exercise, even if you're not feeling fearful or anxious at that moment. If the fear occurs anytime later, you should repeat the relaxation exercise again.

# 11

# PHARMACOLOGICAL
# INTERVENTIONS

Psychotherapeutic drugs aren't like antibiotics; they don't eradicate the causes of anxiety or depression. They work more in the way that insulin does with diabetes; they are often effective in controlling symptoms so that a patient can return to his normal level of functioning. They do so by lifting the heavy darkness of depression, reducing obsessive thoughts, and allowing a parent to perceive fears and worries more realistically.

Seniors are generally more sensitive instruments whose drug use must be more carefully and cautiously monitored. A dose of Prozac is more likely to produce side effects in your eighty-year-old mother than you. Physiological changes in her body can result in different rates of drug absorption, metabolism, storage, and sensitivity. These alterations can result in drugs taking more time to be effective, producing unique or stronger side effects, or remaining in her system longer. If she is suffering from memory problems as well, she is less likely to take the drug as prescribed or to report troublesome side effects.

These are all reasons why it's important for you to understand the special issues regarding medication use in late life before your parent embarks on a prescription-drug regimen for an anxiety disorder.

This is an area where you can be a real help and advocate. By helping a parent understand a drug and its effectiveness, informing the doctor about chronic illnesses, allergies, and other medicines your parent is taking, keeping track of prescriptions and dosages, and watching for side effects, you can help your parent remain safely and effectively on treatment.

# BENEFITS OF PHARMACOLOGICAL TREATMENT IN LATE-LIFE ANXIETY

■ Provides more rapid relief from physical distress and symptoms.

■ Works better alone for moderate-severe anxiety or depression than psychotherapy alone. (For mild depression, psychotherapy is equivalent or better.)

■ Easy to administer, often in one dose a day.

■ Fewer clinician visits.

■ Effective for those reluctant to become involved in psychological counseling or treatment.

■ Can be prescribed by a primary-care physician who is not skilled in counseling.

■ Can be maintained for years, if necessary.

## What a Parent—and You—Should Understand When a Doctor Is Prescribing a Drug

■ Why is this drug being prescribed?

■ When might the first signs of improvement be noted?

■ How long before the full benefit of the drug will be felt?

■ How should I feel when the drug is working?

■ What initial side effects can I expect? Can I expect these to fade or persist over time?

■ What long-term side effects might I experience?

■ Is there any nonmedication approach that might be helpful for this condition, either in conjunction with the medicine or instead of it?

■ How long is it necessary to take this medication?

■ What time of day should I take the medicine?

■ Is there a way to simplify the dosage schedule—so that I can take the drug once a day, for example, instead of twice?

■ Do I need to restrict my diet while I'm on this medication? Are there foods (grapefruit, dairy, etc.) I should avoid?

■ Can I drink alcohol while I'm taking this drug?

■ Should the drug be taken in any special way or at a particular time—with food or first thing in the morning, for example?

■ Given the other medicines I'm currently taking, are there any contraindications or drug-drug interactions I should be aware of?

■ Given my current medical condition, are there any special issues?

■ Are there any tests I should have to monitor long-term effects or damage—for example liver enzymes, or EKGs?

■ Will my progress be monitored through regular visits?

■ Is there a particular protocol for getting off the drug—such as gradual tapering? Will the doctor monitor this?

# ISSUES TO CONSIDER WITH MEDICATIONS IN LATE LIFE

## DIFFERENCES IN DRUG ABSORPTION AND ACTION

There is always individual variability in how people react to any particular drug. One patient's anxiety and depression may be lifted by a medication that causes agitation, stomach distress, and insomnia in another.

However, with the elderly, age-related physiological differences must be taken into account, since they can alter the way drugs are metabolized. For example, decreases in enzymatic liver function and kidney filtration affect the processing and elimination of drugs, elevating their concentration in plasma and extending their effects. Due to such changes, many drugs are more slowly metabolized. Antidepressants and benzodiazepines in particular may have less of an initial effect, but once they take hold, the duration of their action lasts longer.[1]

Seniors may also be more sensitive to the cardiovascular and sedative effects of drugs. In the case of benzodiazepines like Valium, Dalmane, Halcyon, and Xanax, falling and memory problems can develop. Side effects often are felt sooner in the elderly, but they can also take longer to appear.

In order to take these changes into account, I usually prescribe a lower dosage of medicine, then increase the dose slowly over time, if necessary— "start low, go slow" is the motto.

My patient Marjorie's social phobia made her resistant to visiting a doctor to discuss her symptoms. Because of this, she decided to use Xanax that had been previously prescribed for her daughter. Since the drug had been helpful for her daughter's occasional jitteriness, Marjorie didn't bother reading the drug insert or dosage precautions and began taking it several times a day, often with alcohol.

This medication had a much more powerful effect on her than her middle-aged daughter and made her unsteady on her feet, dizzy and groggy. Her alcohol use exacerbated these symptoms until one evening she fell in her apartment, hit her head on a table, and was unconscious for several hours before her daughter found her.

Unfortunately, this kind of story is one I hear far too often with the anxious elderly. Mixing and sharing drugs is never a good idea; a medication that works for one person may be ineffective or dangerous for another. Sharing medication is especially hazardous in late life, when the chances of adverse effects grow even higher.

## Noncompliance with Treatment Regimen

Memory problems and cognitive difficulty increase the likelihood that medicines will be taken at the wrong time or at the incorrect dosages.

A study conducted by the Meyers Primary Care Institute found that elderly patients who were made ill by their prescription medicines often took the wrong dosage, took other people's pills, or continued taking medicine after they were told to stop.[2]

"Half the time I can't remember if I took my medicine or not," my patient Jim told me. "So I just double up and take another to make sure."

Psychiatric drugs are not benign; each has its own precautions and contraindications. For example, alcohol should not be mixed with benzodiazepines or antidepressants; slow-release drugs such as Wellbutrin SR should not be broken in two or crushed, while other drugs may be halved. MOAIs cannot be taken with certain foods and beverages. Many psychiatric drugs, such as Paxil, need to be tapered off gradually or new symptoms may appear.

It's important for a patient to be made aware of these precautions and indications when the drug is first prescribed. Small print and technical jargon can discourage patients from reading drug labeling once they have the prescription at home. That's why asking the doctor the questions listed on pages 170–171 can help avoid problems.

## DRUG INTERACTIONS

The Meyers Primary Care Study showed that nearly half of Americans over sixty-five took five or more medicines. This high rate of drug use greatly increases the chances of drug interactions. A parent may also be self-medicating with over-the-counter remedies, herbal remedies, and vitamins, all of which can cause complex effects.

Your parent may be unaware of the reactions drugs can cause or may not report the medications he is already taking that were prescribed by another physician. This is why it's essential that an up-to-date record of all medicines and dosages be supplied to each doctor he visits.

**Drug-drug interactions** can result in unique side effects that differ from those that result from taking the drug alone. For example, taking a tranquilizer such as Valium with an antihistamine may increase drowsiness and make driving dangerous.

Some experts charge that too many pharmacists fail to protect consumers against potentially dangerous interactions of prescription drugs. Some of these effects are serious. For example, monoamine oxidase inhibitors (MAOIs) should not be combined with other antidepressants except under close supervision, and a period of at least four weeks must pass before switching from an MAOI to a non-MAOI antidepressant.

**Drug-food interactions** result when a drug such as an MAOI inhibitor is taken with such foods as cheese or avocados, which contain tyramine that can dangerously increase blood pressure. Grapefruit juice is another food that should not be mixed with some drugs because the juice affects the enzymes that metabolize certain medication.

John discovered that his disoriented mother, Jane, had been going to one specialist after another for her generalized anxiety symptoms, gathering prescription medicines as she went. When he was cleaning out his mother's drawer one afternoon, he discovered a cache of medications that his mother had been mixing and matching like jewelry.

"Where'd you get all this?" he asked her.

His mother was indignant. "My doctors gave them to me," she insisted. Since these prescriptions had all been written for her by physicians—albeit a great number of them—she assumed that they must be safe and that they could be taken together.

## REPORTING OF SIDE EFFECTS

Seniors are less likely to ask about side effects or complain if they experience them. Psychiatric drugs can cause adverse reactions in the elderly that are much less likely in the general population—including low blood pressure and memory loss. Many antidepressants and all benzodiazepines can contribute to unsteadiness and sedation that may result in falls and fractures.

"I didn't want to bother Dr. James about my nausea; I thought I just had a bug or something," a patient named Flora admitted after giving up on Lexapro after only a week. But the side effects of antidepressants such as Lexapro sometimes resolve after several weeks. If Flora had talked to her doctor, she might have given the drug more time, or he might have altered the dose or tried another drug.

This lack of assertiveness is common with older patients who are used to treating doctors as authority figures not to be questioned or bothered. Also, the very nature of anxiety disorders, such as panic disorder or social phobia, can compound a patient's difficulty in speaking up or questioning his medicines.

And there's another important reason why reporting side effects is crucial. Adverse effects can discourage a patient from continuing a medication that is important for her health or getting a replacement medication. Flora's negative experience with Lexapro makes it less likely that she will try another drug in the future for her depression and anxiety.

## CHRONIC ILLNESS AND PREEXISTING HEALTH CONDITIONS

These can complicate the effectiveness of drugs and may even make them potentially harmful. Each drug has special indications for preexisting health conditions. A patient who has liver disease or a history of alcohol dependence should not be prescribed benzodiazepines. Beta-blockers such as Inderal, used in treating performance anxiety, slow the heart rate and should not be used with people who have certain cardiac problems. MAOIs aren't recommended for those with high blood pressure, epilepsy, cardiac problems, or asthma.

This is another reason why it's essential that any new doctor a parent visits should have a full medical history before another drug is prescribed.

## STIGMA ASSOCIATED WITH PSYCHIATRIC DRUGS

Older people tend to be more skeptical of psychological treatment in general. Taking a pill to help their depressed or anxious mood may seem frivolous, even sinful, to a parent who was brought up before the advent of commonly used psychiatric medications. Parents may also harbor the belief that drugs should only be used for dire physical illnesses.

Common responses in late life include:

"I can handle it myself. I've never taken pills in my life and I'm not taking any now," as one patient told me. But many anxiety and depressive disorders are extremely hard to counter without medication. Your parent needs to be reassured that it's not a sign of weakness to take medication to cope with an anxiety disorder.

"I'm scared of being drugged and groggy. I don't want to be all drugged up like some zombie," as another patient said. "This is my personality and I just have to live with it." Unlike many older drugs that were likely to make a patient feel dulled or sedated, newer drugs such as the SSRIs are often able to lift depression, stabilize mood, and make a patient feel more like herself without adverse effects.

"I don't want to become hooked on a drug." Most medications recommended for late life, such as the SSRIs and BuSpar, do not produce cravings the way older benzodiazepines did. A person will not develop the "urge" to take more Prozac as he might Valium, Xanax, or alcohol. However, it is generally recommended that medications be tapered off gradually whenever a patient stops taking them.

## COMMON MEDICATIONS FOR ANXIETY AND DEPRESSION

### Serotonin Reuptake Inhibitors (SSRIs)

Older drugs such as Valium and Librium may have been developed specifically to target anxiety, but it's now widely accepted that the best class of medicines for all anxiety disorders is the SSRIs, which were initially developed as antidepressants.

Research strongly suggests that the neurotransmitters serotonin, dopamine, GABA, and norepinephrine are disordered in people with anxiety

## Common Features of All SSRIs

■ Work by boosting serotonin reuptake; some also boost other neuro-transmitters

■ Most can be taken once daily

■ Have lower risks of serious adverse reactions, if taken in overdose, than older medications

■ Most commonly caused side effects include: nausea, dizziness, constipation, headache, insomnia, nervousness, tremors, weight gain, and sexual dysfunction

■ Require at least two and up to eight weeks to realize full effectiveness

■ Should be withdrawn from gradually, under doctor's supervision

■ Are contraindicated for patients taking tricyclics or MAOIs (monoamine oxidase inhibitors)—at least four weeks must pass before switching to these drugs

■ Should be used very cautiously by those who suffer from kidney and liver disease

■ May require lower dosage in elderly

disorders and depression. SSRI drugs increase the availability of serotonin, the chemical messenger in the brain that has been shown to regulate pain, anxiety, and pleasure. Some SSRIs also boost other neurotransmitters, such as norepinephrine.

SSRIs are the drugs prescribed first for older people because they are better tolerated; they usually require a single daily dose and have fewer and less troublesome side effects than older drugs.

It's important for patients to understand the complexities of these drugs and how they work. For example, a person won't feel immediately more relaxed or in a better mood after beginning SSRIs. It can take up to eight weeks for the full effects of these medications to become apparent. The first symptom to improve might be sleep or appetite, rather than anxiety or depression. Unlike Valium or related drugs, your parent *must continue* taking these drugs even when he feels better. Seniors who do not realize this may give up too early, before the medicine has "kicked in," or stop it right after feeling better.

"My mother has taken every antidepressant in the book—for about six months," a daughter of a senior woman told me. "As soon as her mood improves, she stops. Then, when it plummets again, she goes back to the doctor and asks for another one."

Another reason why a parent should remain on SSRIs for an adequate period is that certain minor side effects abate after several weeks. Another daughter reported to me: "My dad had insomnia and restlessness for the first two weeks on Paxil, but the doctor had told him to expect it, and so he stuck it out. By the third week, almost all the effects had disappeared and he felt much better. . . ."

Some seniors are so anxious and confused that they don't even remember what the doctor tells them about special features of their prescription drugs. Or they may feel unable to understand the technical small print of contraindications and warnings that accompany them. That's why it's extremely helpful if you can accompany your parent on doctor visits when drugs are being prescribed.

If side effects such as nausea, insomnia, dizziness, or disorientation develop, a parent should always notify the doctor. But he should also be prepared to "stick it out" for a week or two if the doctor feels the side effects are mild. In addition, even when one SSRI doesn't work, another one might. Or the doctor may raise the dosage or add another medication to boost it. Parents and doctors need to be creative and persistent in finding the unique treatment regimen that works.

SSRIs should be tapered off slowly, under a doctor's guidance, to prevent the return of symptoms or the development of new ones. These drugs vary in their half-lives—the amount of time required for the body to eliminate one half of the drug. With Prozac, for example, significant levels remain in the body for several weeks. On the other hand, with Paxil, blood levels drop very quickly, and withdrawal symptoms can develop if the medication is abruptly stopped.

Because of the risk and potential for withdrawal problems, a patient should never stop taking a psychiatric drug or begin taking a new one without a doctor's guidance.

# SSRIs

**Brand name:** Prozac (Fluoxetine)
**Approved for:** Depression, OCD
**Special features:**
First SSRI on market
Extended half-life, remains in system longer than other SSRIs
May initially cause activating symptoms of increased anxiety

**Brand name:** Celexa (Citalopram)
**Approved for:** Depression
**Special features:**
Has a chemical structure unrelated to that of other SSRIs or of tricyclic, tetracyclic, or other available antidepressant agents

**Brand name:** Lexapro (Escitalopram)
**Approved for:** Depression with anxiety; also has shown effectiveness for panic disorder, social anxiety disorder, and GAD
**Special features:**
Newest SSRI. Lexapro is a "purer" form of Celexa.

**Brand name:** Paxil (Paroxetine)
**Approved for:** Depression, GAD, social anxiety disorder, panic disorder, obsessive-compulsive disorder, and posttraumatic stress disorder
**Special features:**
Nausea side effect can be reduced by taking with food
Possible withdrawal effects make it crucial to wean off Paxil gradually. An extended-release formulation makes this less of a concern.

**Brand name:** Zoloft (Setraline)

**Approved for:** Depression, social anxiety disorder, OCD, PTSD, panic disorder

**Special features:**

Safer for those with renal failure and cardiac problems

Diarrhea and weight gain side effects

# OTHER ANTIANXIETY AND ANTIDEPRESSANT MEDICATIONS

**Brand name:** Effexor (Venlafaxine)

**Approved for:** Depression, social anxiety disorder, GAD

**Benefits:** May have fewer side effects than other antidepressants. Effexor has a chemical makeup different from other antidepressants. It is called a SSNRI, a selective serotonin and norepinephrine reuptake inhibitor, because it boosts both of these neurotransmitters.

**Side effects:** Nausea, headache, sleepiness, dry mouth, dizziness, insomnia, constipation, sexual dysfunction. May cause increase in blood pressure.

**Precautions:** Cannot be taken concurrently with monoamine oxidase inhibitors (MAOIs) or within at least fourteen days of discontinuing use.

Effexor XR is an extended-release form of the drug and requires only once-a-day dosing. Nausea, a common side effect, often resolves within a week.

Because of possible elevation, blood pressure should be monitored in the elderly, especially at the beginning of treatment. Withdrawal from the drug also requires careful and gradual tapering, so discontinuation symptoms don't occur.

**Brand name:** Wellbutrin, Zyban (Bupropion)

**Approved for:** Depression, smoking cessation

**Benefits:** No sexual dysfunction or weight gain; safer for patients who have cardiac problems

**Side effects:** Headache, sleep difficulties, insomnia, dry mouth; higher likelihood of causing seizures than other antidepressants.

**Precautions:** Due to slight seizure risk, dosages should remain below 450 mg. Not recommended for anyone with seizure disorder, epilepsy, anorexia, or heavy alcohol use. Cannot be used with MAOIs.

Unrelated to any other antidepressant, Wellbutrin is a unicyclic; the mechanism of its effectiveness involves boosting both the serotonin and dopamine systems. It is also available in extended release (XR) and sustained release (SR) forms.

Wellbutrin is less likely to cause weight gain or sexual dysfunction than the SSRIs and is believed by some to increase libido rather than lessen it. Wellbutrin is sometimes used by clinicians to "boost" the effectiveness of SSRIs or to counteract their sexual side effects.

**Brand name:** BuSpar (buspirone)

**Approved for:** Chronic anxiety, GAD

**Side effects:** Dizziness, headaches, nausea, insomnia

**Benefits:** Nonaddictive, few side effects. Does not potentiate alcohol

BuSpar possesses a number of qualities that make it suitable for use in the elderly. While not as fast-acting as the benzodiazepines, it also doesn't have their negative qualities. It does not cause the sedation, addiction, or cognitive impairment problems associated with benzodiazepines. As a result, it has a significantly lower abuse potential and no withdrawal problems. It can also be used when a parent has preexisting medical conditions.

BuSpar can be helpful in treating late-life chronic anxiety and GAD. The side effects of stomach distress, dizziness, and fatigue can often be mitigated by raising the dose slowly and having the patient take the medicine with meals. BuSpar takes several weeks for its full effects to be felt, so it cannot be used on an as-needed basis. It may not be as effective as the benzodiazepines.

## BETA-BLOCKERS

**Brand name:** Inderal (propranolol)
**Approved for:** Performance anxiety, panic attacks
**Benefits:** Rapid effectiveness, not habit-forming
**Side effects:** Slows heart rate, reduces blood pressure
**Precautions:** Should not be used by people with slow pulse rate

Beta-blockers block the physical manifestations of performance anxiety and panic attacks—heart palpitations, shaking, and sweating—effectively reducing the adrenaline rush and hyperarousal symptoms that are features of these disorders. They are fast-acting and nonaddictive, but lower doses may be necessary in the elderly. Because they slow the heart rate and reduce blood pressure, caution should be used with those who have other health conditions, such as certain cardiac problems, diabetes, asthma, or vascular disease.

"I thought I'd have to give up playing the clarinet in our community orchestra because my performance anxiety was so out of control," my patient James told me. "My heart beat so fast I felt like I was going to faint. There were several occasions when I had to leave the stage and go home. But now I take the beta-blocker you prescribed an hour before our concerts and I feel relaxed. It's amazing what a difference this medicine has made."

## TRICYCLICS (TCAs) AND TETRACYCLICS

**Brand names:** Adapin, Anafranil, Asendin, Elavil, Janimine, Ludiomil, Pamelor, Pertofrane, Sinequan, Surmontil, Tofranil, Vivactil
**Approved for:** Acute depression, panic, GAD, PTSD, OCD
**Benefits:** Nonaddictive, usually require single daily dose

**Side effects:** Can affect heart rhythm and lower blood pressure (hypotensive effects). Drop in blood pressure may lead to falls and fractures. Also frequently causes weight gain, sedation, tremors, twitches, constipation, blurred vision, urinary retention, weight gain, and forgetfulness. Very dangerous when taken in overdose.

**Precautions:** Can be affected by many other drugs, including SSRIs, and can potentiate effects of alcohol. May not be used with MAOIs.

The TCAs and tetracyclics are an older class of antidepressants that have proven effective for treating severe depression, but their numerous side effects have led most doctors to abandon their use.

The tricyclic antidepressant Elavil tops the list of drugs that are counterindicated for use with elderly patients because of their serious side effects. One study in South Dakota found that Elavil was the most inappropriately prescribed medication for the elderly.[3]

I still use the tricyclic Pamelor (nortriptyline) for a patient who has severe depression that has not responded to other medications, since it can be monitored and measured in the blood to discern the effective level.

Though some of these drugs' troublesome effects abate over time, the possibility of cardiac difficulties and sedation, and the increased risk of falls and injuries, combine to make them useful only as a last resort, when others fail to work.

"My mother fell twice when she was on Elavil and then the same thing happened on Ludomil," a daughter of a nursing-home patient reported. "The second time she broke her hip, and she has never really recovered. A fracture when you're over eighty is a serious setback. I wish I'd paid attention earlier to the side effects of her medication."

# BENZODIAZEPINES

**Brand names:** Ativan, Xanax, Valium, Centrax, Dalmane, Diazepam, Doral, Halcion, Klonopin, Librium, Paxilpam, ProSom, Restoril, Serax, Tranxene

**Approved for:** Panic, social anxiety, GAD, insomnia

**Benefits:** Rapid results can be felt within first day

**Side effects:** Drowsiness, dizziness, cognitive impairment; should be careful driving or using machinery; mild amnesia, impairment of physical coordination. Habit-forming, must be tapered off. Should not be mixed with alcohol.

**Precautions:** Should be used with caution in patients with pulmonary, hepatic, and renal disease or history of alcohol and drug dependence or abuse.

In the late 1960s, these drugs replaced older, more dangerous barbiturates and opiates, which slowed breathing and could easily cause death by overdose. These drugs were once the first-line treatment of choice for anxiety, and are still very popular, with Xanax and Valium expressly approved for treating anxiety disorders.

For seniors, I only prescribe these medications for occasional, short-term use at a low dosage when a patient is undergoing a traumatic or severely anxious life event—for example, for a claustrophobic patient who needs to undergo an MRI scan, or a newly widowed woman who is having panic attacks in the wake of her husband's death. Very occasionally I will prescribe them for a person with chronic anxiety, but only if all else has failed.

It's not that these medications aren't effective; they are. Drugs such as Xanax and Ativan are fast-acting, often working in as little as an hour to slow brain activity, and are especially effective for anxiety disorders that require rapid remediation, such as panic.

But their side effects, especially falls, sedation, and amnesia, can be so problematic for older people that I discourage their use. Sedation and coordination problems may be troublesome for a young adult, but for an older person with frail bones it can be far more serious.

Daily use of antianxiety drugs in the young and old can also lead to physical dependence over time. Like alcohol and barbiturates, these drugs induce changes in the brain that lead to craving. It is easy for elderly parents to become reliant on drugs such as Xanax,

Ativan, or Valium, and to find themselves unable to sleep or relax without them.

The benzodiazepines differ sharply in their half lives, and this also affects the side-effect profile. For example, Ativan has a short half-life; any single pill lasts for up to fifteen hours. Klonopin, on the other hand, is far longer-acting, with an average half-life close to one hundred hours. This is relevant, since if a patient stops Ativan, he's much more likely to experience withdrawal symptoms than if he had been taking Klonopin. In general, shorter-acting drugs, such as Lorazepam, are a better idea for the elderly than longer-acting ones, such as Diazepam or Klonopin. When I prescribe these medications for an older patient, I always prescribe lower doses because of the risk of unwanted outcomes.

Withdrawal from these drugs can result in more anxiety symptoms, including panic, shakiness, and insomnia. Severe symptoms may include confusion and seizures. Due to their slower metabolisms, the elderly might not experience withdrawal for a week or even longer. Withdrawal from these drugs can be life-threatening.

## ANTIPSYCHOTICS

**Brand names:** Haldol, Zyprexa, Risperdol, Seroquel, Abilify, Prolixin, Clozaril

**Approved for:** Psychosis (hallucinations and delusions). Used to treat agitation and aggression associated with dementia and certain brain injuries. Occasionally used to treat severe depression. I recommend against their use for anxiety unless it occurs with other symptoms.

**Side effects:** Abnormal involuntary movements similar to Parkinson's disease, which sometimes become permanent; sedation; weight gain; gastrointestinal distress; cardiac arrythmias; elevated blood sugar

**Precautions:** May cause depression and lack of coordination

The wide range of potentially hazardous effects that can impact the elderly make the antipsychotics useful only in special situations

where anxiety or depression is accompanied by delusions or hallucinations.

These drugs were originally developed to treat schizophrenia and
have been a boon to people with this severe mental illness. The newer
drugs (Abilify, Geodon, Seroquel, Zyprexa, Risperdol) cause fewer side
effects than the older ones, especially tardive dyskinesia, a disorder that
results in repetitive, often permanent involuntary movements. However, even these newer antipsychotics have serious side effects and can
cause elevated blood sugar (diabetes), substantial weight gain, and with
one drug, Clozaril, risk of a deadly blood disorder.[4]

# MONOAMINE OXIDASE
# INHIBITORS (MAOIs)

**Brand names:** Nardil, Parnate, Marplan, Eldepryl
**Approved for:** Resistant, chronic depression; depression with anxiety;
  social anxiety; phobias; panic
**Side effects:** Insomnia, weight gain, sluggishness, increased blood pressure
**Precautions:** Restricted diet, limiting cheese, chocolate, red wine, aged
  meat products. Cannot be used with decongestants or other antidepressants. Not advised for those with cardiac problems, high blood
  pressure, asthma, or epilepsy.

Monoamine oxidase inhibitors (MAOIs) work by boosting three
transmitters—serotonin, norepinephrine, and dopamine. Some experts
consider Nardil (phenelzine) the drug of choice for phobias and to be
particularly effective for social anxiety. But due to the cardiovascular effects and restricted diet associated with these drugs, I only use them as a
last resort, when a patient with resistant depression doesn't respond to
other medications.

The dietary restrictions that are necessary in order to safely take
these drugs require medical management and can be cumbersome for

an elderly patient to monitor. MAOIs require a diet that rules out a wide array of foods and beverages, including wine, cheese, beer, aged foods, raisins, soy sauce, chicken liver, and overripe bananas. These foods all contain tyramine, a substance that in combination with MAOIs can cause a dangerous increase in blood pressure. The results of this can be so severe that blood vessels in the brain may burst.

The complexity of these food restrictions can be too much for a younger person, let alone an elderly one with memory problems. Mary, eighty-six, who had been placed on MAOIs after other antidepressants failed, found the food monitoring too much. "It was so confusing. Most cheeses were forbidden, but cream cheese and cottage cheese were allowed. The doctor said I could have a small amount of chocolate now and then, but I never knew how much was too much. I was always nervous when I went out to eat that something forbidden was included in the food. It wasn't worth it."

Mary had to wait over a month before she could switch to another antidepressant, since MAOIs require at least a four-week "washout" period before another drug can be tried. If switching from a long-lasting drug like Prozac, as many as five to eight weeks must pass.

# HERBS AND SUPPLEMENTS FOR ANXIETY AND DEPRESSION

Dietary supplements, herbs, and vitamins are not held to the same strict standards that the FDA has set up for prescription medicines, meaning they are often not studied for either efficacy or safety. Variations in quality, purity, strength, and dosing requirements make them difficult to monitor, and each has its own set of precautions. None of these facts, however, has kept them from being widely used.

Although I make little use of these remedies in my practice, I know that they are attractive because they are natural, and many people claim they are effective in allaying anxiety, especially for patients who cannot tolerate or do not wish to take prescription drugs.

Following are the most commonly used anxiety and depression remedies, herbs, and supplements. Given the large number of drugs most elderly patients take, it is important that these supplements be discussed first with a patient's primary doctor to make sure that there are no contraindications with existing illnesses or currently prescribed medications.

### SAM-e

**Effective for:** Depression, arthritis, fibromyalgia, migraine
**Benefits:** Few side effects, fast-acting
**Side effects:** Stomach upset
**Precautions:** SAM-e should not be taken with phenelzine sulfate or tranylcypromine sulfate or by those suffering from bipolar disorder

A dietary supplement that has been used in Europe since 1975 as an antidepressant, SAM-e stands for S-adenosylmethionine, which consists of two amino acids that are naturally occurring substances in the body. These substances have been reported to be low in patients suffering from depression and other conditions.

SAM-e reportedly works by increasing levels of serotonin, dopamine, and phosphatidylserine without the side effects of some prescription drugs. Other studies claim that it soothes arthritis, fibromyalgia, migraine symptoms, and liver ailments.[5]

However, these studies generally did not include those with moderate or severe depression or anxiety, and many were not appropriately designed.

### St. John's Wort (*Hypericum perforatum*)

**Effective for:** Mild depression, anxiety, insomnia, GAD
**Benefits:** Well-tolerated, few side effects or adverse reactions
**Side effects:** Gastrointestinal distress, sun sensitivity, constipation, dizziness
**Precautions:** Should not be combined with other antidepressant, anti-anxiety, or anticoagulant medications. Since it may enhance bleeding, it should not be used for a week prior to surgery.

One of the most commonly used antidepressants in Germany, St. John's wort has a long history as a nerve soother. European studies have reported that it is an antidote for mild depression, anxiety, and stress. Its reported effects are based on its stabilizing influence on serotonin and dopamine, similar to prescription SSRIs. It may take up to four weeks for full effects to be felt, and it may interfere with the function of other drugs. A recent review concluded that it was not effective for moderate or severe depression.

### Valerian

**Effective for:** Anxiety, insomnia
**Benefits:** Fast-acting, no morning hangover effect
**Side effects:** Gastrointestinal upset, sleepiness
**Precautions:** Should not be mixed with antianxiety or sedative drugs

In Europe, valerian is a well-known sleep aid that also produces a generally calming effect. In studies of insomniacs, valerian was reported to be as effective as prescription sedatives in inducing sleep, with a reduction in morning grogginess. It appears to work by influencing brain receptors for the neurotransmitter GABA. There is no good evidence that it is effective for anxiety or depression.

### Kava Kava (*Piper methysitcum*)

**Benefits:** Fast-acting, nonaddictive
**Effective for:** Anxiety, insomnia, panic, restlessness, muscle relaxant
**Side effects:** Gastrointestinal upset, allergic skin reaction
**Precautions:** Can cause psychosis, neurological and severe liver damage

Kava has been reported to reduce such anxiety symptoms as nervousness, heart palpitations, and sleeplessness.

Even though a review of several double-blind studies looking at the effectiveness of kava for anxiety symptoms suggested the superiority of it over placebo, I believe it is too dangerous. Because of the liver damage it can cause, which may lead to the need for a liver transplant, I do not recommend that it be used at all.

## HOW YOU CAN HELP

■ Accompany your parent on medical visits when drugs are being prescribed or discussed—or find someone who can do it for you.

■ Whenever a parent visits a new doctor, assist him by bringing along all medications, including over-the-counter remedies, that he is currently taking, so an accurate medical record can be made.

■ Monitor a parent's symptoms, even those that might not seem central to anxiety or depression. Sometimes you will be the one who notices that he seems more active or less negative, even when he claims he feels unchanged. This can be helpful to the doctor and may help your parent remain in treatment.

■ Monitor your parent's medications; ask weekly about side effects. Provide your parent with a special notebook for noting drug reactions and symptom levels.

■ When a parent is taking multiple drugs, make sure the labels are clearly marked and easy to read.

■ Obtain seven-day weekly pill dividers to ensure a parent takes the correct daily dose.

■ Make sure the medication your parent is receiving is correct. Doctor and pharmacist errors are as responsible as patient errors for prescription drug problems.

■ Reevaluate with the doctor whether a parent's medication should be continued after symptoms have abated. Some psychiatric drugs may not be needed for an extended period.

■ Clear out a parent's medicine cabinet of drugs that have expired.

## COMMON DOSES OF ANXIETY
## MEDICATIONS FOR ELDERLY

| | |
|---|---|
| Zoloft | 25–150 mg per day |
| Paxil | 5–40 mg per day |
| Effexor | 75–300 mg per day, starting off at 37.5 mg |
| Prozac | 5–20 mg per day |
| Celexa | 10–20 mg per day |
| Lexapro | 10–20 mg per day |
| Xanax | .25 mg, 1 to 3 times per day |
| Valium | 5–20 mg per day |
| Ativan | 0.5 mg, 1 to 3 times a day |
| Klonopin | 0.25 mg, 1 to 2 times a day |

# 12

# CALMING THERAPIES

Your mother is in a crowded bus stuck in traffic in the Midtown Tunnel, when suddenly she experiences the onset of a panic attack. She feels sweaty, closed in, and apprehensive—the way she did when she was involved in a bus accident last year. In fact, the sensations are so intense that they feel like a flashback to that earlier event when she was trapped and felt unable to breathe. And just like in the earlier event, there is no room for her to change seats or open a window. The Xanax her doctor gave her for such emergencies is in her medicine chest at home; she doesn't have a cell phone to call you or your sister. She's left to her own devices for the duration of the trip.

Is there anything she can do to calm herself and head off a full-blown anxiety attack in such a situation? The answer is unequivocally *yes*.

Even in the middle of harrowing conditions there are a variety of calming methods that can be self-administered to help banish attacks of panic and anxiety.

The beauty of these techniques is that they require no prescription, special skills, or equipment. They can also be used anywhere—at the grocery store, when an attack of agoraphobia sets in; on the stage, when a bout of performance anxiety appears; in the hospital waiting room, before a stressful medical test.

Techniques such as deep breathing, meditation, progressive muscle relaxation, yoga, and tai chi are all particularly beneficial with late-life anxiety and may be used in conjunction with each other, pharmacological treatments, or psychotherapy.

These calming techniques promote serenity and a sense of empowerment and control at a time when so many other aspects of independence may be diminishing. They can also be employed in group settings, providing structure and companionship as well as relaxation.

These skills are assets that can be used throughout life. In fact, they can be as beneficial for *you* as your anxious parent. These calming techniques and serenity skills can be of mutual benefit, and can be jointly learned and utilized.

Sara, the daughter of an anxious mother, told me: "I was playing my mother a relaxation tape the other day when all of a sudden it dawned on me that *I* needed this as much as she did. In my rush to make sure she's okay—along with everyone else in my family—I'm a frazzled wreck half the time, and lately my blood pressure's gone through the roof. Sharing this with her is not only a nice interlude and something we can enjoy together, but it's beneficial for both of us. Sometimes I just say to her now, 'C'mon, Mom, let's just close our eyes a minute and do some deep breathing.'"

## TAI CHI

Years ago, on a trip to Japan, I drove by a grassy village square where a group of older adults was congregated, moving in a lovely, choreographed way. Their graceful, spiraling movements were so entrancing that I stopped my car to watch. The participants' faces were intent, their bodies relaxed and fluid. I realized how rarely I saw seniors like this, out in public, engaged in such a beautiful physical display.

They were practicing tai chi, an ancient Eastern art that combines elements of meditation, yoga, and breathing. It's a practice that is growing increasingly popular with older adults who have discovered its power to relax and strengthen their bodies as well as increase flexibility and balance.

Tai chi focuses on deep breathing and gentle, flowing movements. These relaxing moves promote regular breathing and a serene mind. Tai chi is particularly beneficial in late life, since it causes little strain on the body, and by improving balance, coordination, and mobility, it also reduces the risk of falling. Studies have shown a significant improvement in physical functioning in elderly tai chi participants along with a lessening of depression symptoms.[1]

Tai chi classes are traditionally led by an instructor, but students are encouraged to memorize the movements so they can practice them on their own.

One grandmother told me: "No one in my family could believe it when I took up tai chi at seventy-one, but my range of motion is now as good as my daughter's. Whenever I get harried or overwrought, I go out into the backyard and practice my forms. It's also improved my memory and concentration."

## THE POWER OF THE BREATH

Anne, an eighty-two-year-old diabetic patient, developed increasing panic after the death of her husband. She lived alone and was committed to remaining independent. But after several incidents when her insulin levels had wildly fluctuated, she felt so vulnerable and frightened that she had full-blown panic attacks, with difficulty breathing and a rapid, racing heartbeat.

One winter evening, during a snowstorm, she had a particularly severe attack. The weather was treacherous, and she didn't want to call her family or the ambulance for a trip to the emergency room. Then she remembered a breathing technique a friend had taught her when they'd been together on a turbulent flight overseas.

Anne closed her eyes and began breathing slowly from her abdomen—inhaling through her nose and exhaling through pursed lips. She continued to do this, slowly and methodically, and, in half an hour, she had calmed herself enough to get into bed and fall asleep.

Many people don't appreciate how powerful deep breathing can be as a tool for stress reduction, an on-the-spot, simple way to eradicate anxiety symptoms such as Anne's. Deep breathing can both soothe nervous thoughts and overcome anxiety's physical manifestations.

"I like that I don't have to take a pill—that I can do this for myself," Anne said.

When the body is tense, breathing often grows shallow and rapid, contributing to a sensation of smothering and feelings of weakness and panic.

When we're breathing normally, the body senses the carbon dioxide level and adjusts the breathing rate accordingly. When tense, our muscles tighten, and a feeling of smothering leads to rapid breathing, which triggers more discomfort. Since muscles relax during exhalation, one goal of relaxed breathing is to prolong the release of breath.

## Anxiety-Reducing Breath

The following breath is adapted from yogic breathing techniques. This approach involves slow abdominal breathing, with the focus on an elongated exhale.

Sit comfortably with feet flat on the floor and eyes closed.
Exhale completely.
Take a deep, slow breath in through the nose to a count of four.
Feel the stomach grow soft and expand with the deep inhalation.
Slowly release the deep breath and exhale very slowly through the mouth,
    to a count of six. Pull in the stomach to expel all the remaining breath.
Relax and let go, feeling the tension vanish.
Repeat for up to five minutes.

This breath is effective in calming panic and sleeplessness. Patients with phobic disorders can also use it to cope with stressful situations.

### HYPERVENTILATION

Abnormally rapid and often shallow breathing, hyperventilation is common in panic attacks, and results in a variety of physical symptoms, such as dizziness, sighing, yawning, and the sensation of difficulty catching one's breath.

Breathing into a paper bag is a way of counteracting hyperventilation. By recycling the exhaled air, this technique increases levels of carbon dioxide and results in a slower breathing rate and an easing of symptoms.

## BIOFEEDBACK

I had one extremely tense patient who performed her relaxing breaths while using a mirror as a monitor. When performing deep breathing, she looked at her reflection in the mirror and tried to make her face and jaw as relaxed as possible. She found that the more at ease her face felt, the deeper was her total relaxation.

This process is a form of biofeedback, a method that heightens awareness and control of a body function, such as breathing, muscle tension, body temperature, heart rate, or blood pressure, and alters it through relaxation.

Biofeedback is another method seniors can use to develop control over their anxiety symptoms and manage stress. By teaching the mind how it can influence bodily functions, biofeedback can help a patient become aware of the mind-body connection and short-circuit anxiety attacks.

Biofeedback has proven effects in many studies. In one, yoga relaxation methods coupled with biofeedback were effective in lowering blood pressure up to 16 points.[2] Other studies have shown biofeedback's effectiveness in inducing relaxation, reducing tension headaches, and lessening the frequency of other stress-related illnesses.

A typical technique involves attaching a device to a patient's finger, which connects them to a machine that measures skin temperature or perspiration. The machine then produces a signal, such as a beep or a light, whenever tenseness, as measured by a drop in skin temperature or perspiration, is detected. As a result, the patient learns to recognize the sensation of tension and learns how to control it by muscle relaxation.

The goal is for the patient to try different methods to reduce tension and thus extinguish the sound or light. The person might visualize certain tranquil scenes or imagery, perhaps combined with relaxed breathing. Since tensing or becoming more anxious will make the beep louder, or the light brighter, the patient eventually learns through trial and error which methods lessen his anxious state. He thus discovers what his tension "feels" like and what can help him relax it away. This general principle is the basis of all biofeedback methods.

## TYPES OF BIOFEEDBACK

A **galvanic skin response (GSR)** measures the electrical conductance of skin, which is correlated to sweat-gland activity. Tenseness is detected as an increase in the glandular activity that produces sweat. This method is often used for treating anxiety and phobias and is also the method used for lie-detector testing.

An **electromyogram (EMG)** monitors muscle tension. Electrodes are placed on the muscles that need to be monitored such as the shoulders or jaw. The machine emits a signal when the electrodes detect muscle tension.

**Temperature biofeedback** monitors skin temperature and is often used to induce relaxation. A sensor is usually attached to a foot or finger. A drop in skin temperature alerts a patient to lessening tenseness, which he experiences as a lowering of anxiety.

**Electroencephalogram (EEG)** methods monitor brain-wave activity, which emit various frequencies of electrical signals—alpha waves being correlated with a relaxed state.

By learning how to control the internal process of relaxation, a patient becomes able to combat the buildup of tension in daily life situations and head off or abort a panic or anxiety attack.

# MEDITATION

A central component of Buddhist and Hindu worship, the ancient practice of meditation focuses on quieting the mind and body. Meditation is a way of silencing the inner chatter so common to anxiety disorders—whether it's dread of an upcoming social event, fixation on a feared object, or a flashback to a past, stressful event.

By centering the mind on the breath, a thought, or an image, meditation transports a person out of the thicket of anxiety and produces a state of deep relaxation.

Increasingly used as a healing tool in Western medicine, meditation is particularly effective for stress-related conditions. Studies have reported that meditation can help ease anxiety and depression as well as decrease blood pressure, heart rate, and counteract secretions of stress hormones. One study reported that a stress-reduction program involving mindful meditation resulted in increased activity in the left frontal regions of the brains of participants—an area associated with positive mood and a reduction in anxiety.[3]

Meditation is one of the simplest relaxation techniques. It doesn't need to be a big production with special pillows, candles, and spiritual music. All that's really required is a quiet spot, a comfortable position, and a thought, mantra, or sound upon which to focus attention.

Marilyn, a retired teacher, told me: "When I first moved to my retirement community, I was completely frantic. I didn't know anyone, and I felt like a fish out of water. I had already been diagnosed with panic disorder, but my symptoms became much worse. When the leader in Activities suggested meditation one day, we all laughed. But after we did it a few times, I saw that all I really had to do is sit comfortably and focus my mind. It's an easy technique that I can use every day to center and calm myself."

The following is a basic meditation that has the effect of relaxing both the body and the mind. What's important is that you breathe slowly and deeply, and that you become focused on the breathing itself.

## Breath Meditation

- Sit comfortably in a quiet place.
- Place your hands on your knees.
- Close your eyes.
- Take a few calming breaths.
- Relax your body—let everything go.
- Pay attention to your breath as you inhale and exhale.
- Breathe in a natural, easy fashion.
- Don't try to alter the breath, just follow its cycle.
- Continue paying attention to your living breath as it enters and exits your body.
- Don't worry about how you're doing or "try" to do well.
- If your attention wanders, gently bring it back to the breath.
- Alternatively, you may focus on a calming word such as "peace," "God," or "love," repeating it over and over as you exhale.
- Continue sitting in this way, focusing on your breath or your calming word for at least five minutes.

Meditation can become a regular relaxation-inducing practice; try a ten-to-twenty-minute session once a day, preferably first thing in the morning.

# VISUALIZATION

Visualization, a crucial component of many relaxation techniques, is a way of harnessing the potent power of the mind and imagination for calming and soothing purposes. It's a way to redirect and control the mind's images.

Patients often see themselves as vulnerable, tense, and anxious. A steady diet of negative images can poison their outlook and have an influence on the way they behave. If patients view themselves as timid and terrified, they're more likely to act that way.

Dale Carnegie and other inspirational writers have long advocated visualization for encouraging high performance and potential. This method is often used by performers and athletes to reach their goals—a baseball player may see himself hitting a home run, or a golfer a hole in one.

The simplest way to use visualization to rapidly calm an anxious mind is to imagine a serene scene and transport yourself there, by focus and deep breathing. The goal is to "see" in the mind's eye the peaceful beach, the calm forest, or the glittering lake—or whatever is especially relaxing—as in the following example.

## Tropical Visualization

- Sit in a recliner or other comfortable spot.
- Close your eyes.
- Take several deep, calming breaths.
- Visualize a golden staircase.
- Picture it clearly in your mind.
- Now see yourself walking down it very slowly.
- With each step of your descent, notice that you are becoming more and more relaxed.
- When you reach the bottom of the stairs, you are standing before a tropical waterfall cascading into a bottomless pool of blue water.
- See this scene very vividly.
- It is a perfect day in every way.
- The sky is blue and cloudless.
- A soft breeze caresses your face.
- The golden light of the sun bathes you.
- You are part of this perfection.
- Stand and breathe the fragrant air.
- Feel the warmth.
- Listen to the water cascading down.

- You are perfectly safe and serene here.
- Nothing can harm you.
- Breathe and see yourself as strong and calm.
- When you're ready, go up the golden staircase and open your eyes.
- Breathe deeply as you gradually become awake to your surroundings.

This can be your own private, tranquil spot where you return whenever you need to relax and calm yourself.

## SPECIAL VISUALIZATIONS

While in this calming location, more specific visualizations can be performed to erase or ease a problem.

### For a GAD sufferer chronically worried about health

See yourself standing in front of the waterfall, feeling healthy and strong, your body glowing, clear of disease and anxiety.

See any negative emotions or fears drip out of your fingers like black ink and disappear into the ground. Or see your worries as a flock of black birds that fly from your mind and disappear above the waterfall.

### For panic attacks

Visualize your panic as a small bonfire burning in your mind; now douse it with a pail of the cool blue water from the calming pool.

### For phobias

Relax completely into the poolside scene, then picture yourself in the midst of your feared activity—for example, entering an elevator but remaining calm. If you feel yourself getting tense, return to the relaxing site. Go back and forth between the elevator scene and the tropical site.

Another idea is to visualize the feared object or situation as a bright orange cloud in your mind, then slowly change it to the same calming blue as the water in the pool.

You can also combine visualization with relaxation, as in the following exercise for social anxiety.

## For Social Anxiety

1. Identify the most relaxing place you can visualize—for example, sitting on a warm beach with a blue sky and a calm breeze, sitting in a mountain cabin with a view of the mountains from the porch, or sitting on a dock beside a placid pond.
2. Close your eyes and visualize that scene. Really try to get a vivid picture in your mind.
3. While keeping the picture in your mind, relax your arms; start with your fingers and feel the blood flowing through them. Relax the muscles in your hands; then relax your forearms. Do you feel your arms relaxed and getting lighter?
4. Now relax your whole body; continue visualizing the scene, feeling your body relaxing, your arms and legs getting lighter and more relaxed. Now you feel light and relaxed all over.
5. Think about the situation or setting that makes you anxious: the crowded street, the social gathering, or a city bus. As the setting enters your mind, close your eyes and visualize the relaxing scene and think about relaxing your body; then do it again. Do you feel anxious or upset? If yes, repeat.
6. Next think about the situation itself and repeat the visualization of the relaxing scene and the relaxation of your body.

For optimum benefits, visualization should be practiced several times a day—preferably before sleep or first thing in the morning. Repetition is important.

# RELAXATION TECHNIQUES: PROGRESSIVE RELAXATION

Edmund Jacobsen, the psychologist who developed the technique known as progressive relaxation in 1929, believed that the body responded to anxiety and stressful events by producing muscle tension, and that the tension cycled back to further increase anxiety.

To break this cycle, he developed the progressive relaxation technique, which involves tensing then relaxing sets of muscle in order to reduce tension. The idea is that you can voluntarily control muscle relaxation and blood flow. Progressive relaxation has been reported to be effective for stress-related disorders, mild depression, and insomnia. It has also been shown to lead to short-term reductions in pulse, blood pressure, and respiration rates.

In this technique, starting with the feet and moving up the body, each muscle or group of muscles is systematically tensed for five seconds, followed by twenty seconds of relaxation. During the relaxation process, muscles loosen and lead to a sensation of increased blood flow, resulting in a warm, relaxed feeling.

This method can also be shortened and used for specific muscle groups that are particularly tense, such as a stiff neck or shoulder.

## Progressive Relaxation Exercise

- Lie down on your back and close your eyes. Part your feet slightly and place palms up in a receiving position.
- Clear your mind. Close your eyes. Take several deep, calming breaths.
- Tense the muscles of your feet for a count of five. Relax and let go for a count of twenty.
- Tense your calf muscles for a count of five. Relax and let go for a count of twenty.

*(continued)*

- ■ Tense your stomach muscles for a count of five. Relax and let go for a count of twenty.
- ■ Tense your chest muscles for a count of five. Relax and let go for a count of twenty.
- ■ Clench your fists for a count of five. Relax and let go for a count of twenty.
- ■ Tense your neck muscles for a count of five. Relax and let go for a count of twenty.
- ■ Tense your face and head muscles for a count of five. Relax and let go for a count of twenty.

This cycle of relaxation and tension is usually repeated at least once. This exercise can also be done seated upright in a chair.

## YOGA

At a conference last summer, I was standing with a group, and a vibrant woman was the center of attention. She was silver-haired, straight-backed, and elegant, and everyone was turned toward her warming presence. When she moved off, a man next to me said, "How old do you think she is?"

"I don't know," I said. "I'm not good at guessing ages. Sixty, sixty-five?"

"She's eighty-nine," he told me. "Can you believe it? She's a yoga teacher. Maybe we should take it up."

It wasn't just this woman's straight spine and regal bearing that were so impressive. She also had a serenity about her, a look of calm well-being.

I think of her often in my daily practice when I talk with patients who are so caught up with their anxieties and illnesses that they have given up control of everything involved with their body.

An ancient Indian practice, yoga involves a variety of muscle stretches, limbering positions, and controlled breathing exercises that induce relaxation and well-being. Yoga practitioners often speak of how the practice calms their spirits, steadies their minds, and increases vitality. Evidence suggests that practices like yoga and meditation help counteract and reduce anxiety, panic attacks, insomnia, and depression.

Research on a group of sixty-two "stressed" people who underwent a mindfulness-training program that involved yoga postures and meditation reported that thirty-five of them had an average 54 percent reduction in psychological distress—as well as a 46 percent drop in medical symptoms.[4]

Other research focused on women between the ages of sixty-eight and eighty-six who suffered from excessive curvature of the upper spine. Participants attended a one-hour yoga class twice a week for twelve weeks. At the end of the class, not only had the average height of the women increased by half a centimeter along with improvement in spine curvature, but a majority reported a greater sense of well-being and an improvement in physical functioning.[5]

Yoga classes specifically designed for the elderly are now typical offerings in many yoga centers. For the frail elderly, poses can be adapted for lying in bed or sitting in a chair. Safety is key, so make sure you receive instruction from a practitioner who is well trained and knows how to fit the techniques to the special needs of older people.

## Ten Benefits of Yoga in Late Life

- Controls and calms the mind
- Improves posture and balance
- Centers energy
- Aids sleep
- Increases concentration
- Promotes mental and physical harmony
- Increases intake of oxygen through deep breathing
- Keeps joints supple
- Improves circulation
- Increases energy and vitality

## ACCENTUATE THE POSITIVE

A branch of psychological theory called "positive psychology" claims growing evidence that optimists are better off than pessimists in a number of ways. According to Martin Seligman, a researcher and proponent of positive psychology, happy people are healthier, more productive, and more content in their marriages than their unhappy counterparts. Seligman believes that we can control how we think just as we can control our muscles, and that by training the mind to think in a positive fashion, optimism can actually be instilled.

Seligman suggests that someone depressed should try speaking to himself more kindly, the way a dear friend might. The goal is to replace automatic negative thoughts such as "I always mess up, I'm a loser," with a positive alternative, for example: "I had a hard time today, but I gained some insight from my experience that I can use to make tomorrow better."[6]

Teaching the mind to turn in an upbeat direction takes some effort, but with vigilant practice, it can be done. Positive verbal affirmations, such as the following, can help counteract the negative messages that perpetuate anxiety and unhappiness.

- *It is only anxiety; I won't die from it.*
- *I've been through this before and survived.*
- *I am healthy and strong.*
- *Time will pass and so will these feelings*
- *I will not fight these feelings, but experience them.*
- *I will watch my anxiety rise and fall.*
- *I am a survivor.*
- *My anxiety always ends.*
- *I can deal with this.*

# GRATITUDE

Another belief of positive psychology is that those who are grateful for their blessings and count their good fortunes rather than their misfortunes, are generally healthier, happier, and more successful. Rather than their happiness making them grateful, it appears that their being grateful has been the force that has helped make them happy.[7] Experts suggest incorporating gratitude, humor, and generosity into daily interactions with others as a way of fostering fulfillment.

One way to encourage this type of thought is by keeping a gratitude journal, where, each day or week, the patient completes the sentence "Today I am grateful for . . ." then records as much detail as possible. This journal becomes an ever-growing log of good feelings and positive experiences that can provide a sense of comfort and well-being as well as fostering positive thought.

A retired minister, who'd fought depression since the death of his wife, reported: "I spent years focusing on the sadness of my loss, and rarely took stock of all the blessings I still have. Keeping a journal helped me concentrate my attention on the many good things—from my grandchildren to my healthy body—that I'm still lucky enough to possess."

# 13

# LIFESTYLE CHANGES TO COMBAT ANXIETY

Henry, one of my patients with panic, was a man in his seventies who spent his days alone in a dreary garden apartment, eating junk food, watching television, and wandering the night without sleep.

His symptoms were more tenacious and difficult to treat than those of another patient, James. He was suffering from the same disorder, but he got up early to take a brisk walk, ate a balanced meal each day at a local coffee shop with friends, and volunteered at his church.

Social supports, exercise, and a sense of purpose are more crucial than ever in late life, when the structures of work and family have often disappeared, leaving open-ended, empty days. Loneliness, boredom, and inertia are fertile breeding grounds for depression and anxiety.

That's why quality-of-life enhancements, such as physical exercise, nutrition, support groups, volunteering, caring for pets, creativity activities, humor, and spiritual practice are such important ways to enrich and revitalize anxious seniors' lives.

The challenge with older patients is helping them discover the kinds of activities they're authentically interested in, as opposed to what others *think* they should want. Rather than pushing patients in a certain direction, it's more useful to help them rediscover their real interests, as Nancy found out with her depressed father, Jim.

"I tried to get my dad to go to the local senior center for their free lunch, to the synagogue for services, to the health club to exercise, but he shot down every suggestion I made and just stayed at home. Then one night, over dinner, I said: 'Dad, you can do pretty much whatever you want now—what is it you'd really enjoy being involved in?' And he said, without missing a beat, 'Helping kids.'" It was that simple. He'd taught earlier in his life, and it was something he missed. It only took a couple of weeks before we were able to find him a volunteer position in the local school system to mentor at-risk children; it's a regular schedule, which suits him. He really needs structure and regularity. He's much happier and he's doing good at the same time."

Research suggests that most of us are happiest in proximity to others. The human brain seems to have evolved with a need for closeness and intimacy, and functions best with such stimulus.[1] Studies indicate that seniors who remain an involved part of a caring community are better able to flourish into late life.

Some cultures foster this kind of involvement. In a survey of seniors in Okinawa, Japan, many of whom lived alone, less than a third claimed to be lonely. As part of a community that regularly organizes activities for them, Okinawan elders often work far into old age, passing their skills onto younger members. Senior women gain a sense of solace and meaning from a spiritual practice in which they are in charge of saying prayers for the dead. This combination of community care, meaningful work, and spiritual life may be part of the reason why suicide rates in Okinawa are the lowest in East Asia.[2]

Activities that give seniors a sense of focus and purpose can help lessen stress and worry. Hobbies, especially those with a social component, are a way to combine meaningful focus and group interaction. Singing in a chorus, taking part in a sewing circle, book club, or current events discussion group can stimulate the mind and encourage people to mix together, providing a crucial sense of self-definition and engagement.

Dr. Walter Bortz, an associate clinical professor of medicine at Stanford University and author of *Dare to Be 100,* claims that "people who stay involved have a tendency to live longer, as they have more reason to get out of bed in the morning. Their interests stimulate their brains, and this gets their bodies moving."

Bortz practices what he preaches. He and his wife ran the Boston Marathon and became the first married couple in their seventies to finish the race.[3]

## WALKING, NOT ROCKING

When I was growing up, seniors were expected to sit on the sidelines and accept their body's decline. Physical deterioration was believed to be an inevitable part of aging, and exercise was an uncommon activity for older adults. Back then it would have been shocking to see an elderly person jogging or lifting weights.

Luckily, this is an aspect of aging that has improved significantly over the years. Now you're as likely to find seniors in a local health club, riding a stationary bike, as on the front porch in a rocking chair. Today you encounter older adults swimming laps, running marathons, and involved in strength training.

We now realize how vital physical exercise is to optimal aging, how it keeps not only the body supple and limber but also revitalizes the mind and combats anxiety and stress. Studies have long proven the therapeutic benefits of regular exercise in reducing anxiety and depression, increasing longevity and guarding against disease.[4] A fit body is in every way more resilient. Studies have proven that physically active individuals suffer from less stress and associated illness than their inactive counterparts.

**Aerobic exercise,** such as swimming or brisk walking, is a sustained activity of at least twenty minutes that boosts heart rate and respiration. This kind of exercise increases a person's stamina and overall strength.

**Anaerobic exercise,** involving stretching, toning, and weight lifting, is also highly valuable in maintaining flexibility, tone, and balance. Weight training can also help strengthen bones and prevent fractures.

Some type of exercise is possible and beneficial for everyone. Even the frailest, most sedentary elderly can benefit from stretching and strength training. In fact, experts agree that much of the physical decline commonly referred to as "aging" can be prevented or reversed by regular exercise.

---

### Thirteen Ways Exercise Combats Stress and Anxiety in Late Life

1. Produces endorphins, which contribute to elevated mood and increased relaxation
2. Increases levels of serotonin
3. Aids restful sleep
4. Fights depression
5. Boosts self-esteem
6. Banishes worried thoughts
7. Increases sense of well-being
8. Encourages social interaction and contact
9. Reduces blood pressure
10. Aids circulation
11. Helps relax muscles and reduce muscular tension
12. Burns energy released by fight-or-flight response
13. Releases frustration

---

## EXERCISE TIPS FOR SENIORS

**Check with your physician** before you begin exercising, to make sure which type of exercise is safe and beneficial for you. But don't use physical limitations as an excuse. No matter what your condition or age, there is likely some kind of physical activity that will benefit you.

**Ignore old stereotypes.** Resist misconceptions that it's "too late" to exercise, or that exercise might be somehow harmful when you're older. On the contrary, inactivity and lack of initiative are implicated in accelerated aging and many diseases. Loss of muscle mass, or sarcopenia, is now recognized as one of the major contributors to frailty. Regular exercise can help lessen this muscle loss, and the benefits accrue whenever you start. And, amazingly, just eight weeks of exercise can lead to major improvements in strength and lower rates of falling, heart attacks, and stroke.

**Pick an activity you love.** In fact, try to pick one that you don't consider exercise, but pleasure. Walking through a nature preserve, for example, can be a way of enjoying a view of nature along with garnering the benefits of exercise. Or ride a bike to visit a friend.

**Walk!** It doesn't have to be strenuous. A daily brisk walk of twenty or thirty minutes is most beneficial, but you can start out with five minutes twice a week. A dawdling, window-shopping walk, however, won't provide the same benefits.

Dr. Andrew Weil says: "Human beings are made to walk. We are bipedal, upright organisms with bodies designed for locomotion. Walking is a complex behavior that requires functional integration of a great deal of sensory and motor experiences; it exercises our brains as well as our musculoskeletal systems."[5]

**Combine exercise with socializing.** Square dancing at the local community center or joining in a group water-aerobics class is a way of interacting socially with others, which also improves mood and alleviates stress at the same time as you avail yourself of valuable exercise.

**Make it a habit.** Exercise should be a sustained and regular part of your routine. General guidelines suggest exercising for thirty minutes per day four or more days a week. Even two days a week can make a difference, especially if you are already in shape. If you're not fit, sessions should be split into smaller segments and gradually increased in frequency and length.

**Do what you can.** Even if you're sedentary or bedridden, there are stretching, toning, and yoga exercises that can be tailored for you and that can help you retain strength and range of motion.

**It's never too late.** No matter how old you are, exercise has proven benefits. "I never exercised in my life until I was in my seventies," Iris reported. "But when I became depressed after my retirement, I started walking with my neighbor after dinner. It helped my loneliness, I lost weight, and my mood really improved."

## CREATIVITY

Joining groups that foster creativity can expose talents a parent may never have had the time to explore before and open up a new world. Painting, singing, writing, learning a new language, and working with children are all outlets that have a salutary effect, especially when done with other people.

Writing groups, in particular those devoted to reminiscence, can provide a healing, therapeutic sense of life review.

Emily, seventy-two, a retired librarian with multiple sclerosis and agoraphobia, was becoming increasingly isolated and morose. Her daughter bought her a speech-activated computer and enrolled her in a reminiscence-writing class at the local university.

Emily found it gratifying to explore a talent she'd never had time for in the past, and a pleasure to share this work with others. But it was equally important for her to review through her writing all she had accomplished in her life.

"Writing about my life made me reevaluate what I've been through and survived. Sharing my work with a group gave me a way of airing my emotions and worries. I felt less anxious and alone, and I've made new friends."

The process of looking back on a life and putting it on paper seems to provide a reflective catharsis, a sense of the integrity and meaning of one's life. Research shows that this kind of writing can help people handle stress, deal with painful experiences, and increase self-awareness. Studies indicate that it can even be physically therapeutic.

In a study on the health benefits of writing poetry, participants said that writing helped reduce anxiety, cope with the pain of bereavement, and, in some cases, allowed them to stop taking medicines for depression.[6]

Other research found that people with rheumatoid arthritis or asthma who wrote about an emotional experience or the stress in their lives, as opposed to emotionally neutral topics, reduced their symptoms. It's not clear how this occurs, but writing about an upsetting event may interrupt the release of stress hormones that cause anxiety symptoms and can harm the immune system. A single writing exercise eased symptoms for several months.[7]

## SUPPORT GROUPS

At a local VFW hall on a recent Saturday in Nyack, New York, a group of graying men sit in a circle, chatting and drinking coffee, several wearing old army caps and uniforms. This isn't exactly a coffee klatch for elderly vets but a social support that's just as vital to these men, some of whom have been meeting for nearly a decade—a posttraumatic-stress support group. Led by a former veteran and psychologist, group members are encouraged to talk about their feelings and share their common concerns.

Studies show that support groups can dramatically improve psychological well-being and lower rates of anxiety and depression by encouraging group members to discuss their feelings, provide feedback, and promote an atmosphere of trust and candor. Often led by a mental-health professional or other leader, they are a fine way to disseminate information, educate, and share common experiences.

Groups form around shared experiences; the focus may be on shared illnesses, such as diabetes or cancer, or life-changing events such as caregiving or widowhood. These groups foster interaction with others and provide a feeling of camaraderie and support that can be missing from the lives of anxious and isolated elderly.

I've seen the good these groups can do for seniors such as my patient Helen, who developed panic attacks after the death of her husband of fifty years.

"It got so I couldn't drive anymore, I was so panicked, and the medications that calmed me also made me groggy," she said. "I didn't think I would be able to make it on my own. Then my grandson found a grief group sponsored by the local funeral home. There I met a circle of women who'd been through the same thing and were grappling with the same grief I was. Listening to how they survived and coped helped me keep putting one foot in front of the other."

Support groups can be as valuable for a child/caregiver as an anxious parent. A study of Alzheimer's patients found that if you improved the mood of a caregiver you also improved the mood of the person with Alzheimer's.[8] On the other hand, in a study of my own, we discovered that the converse wasn't true: When Alzheimer's patients were treated for depression with medication, the caregiver's mood was unaffected.

My only reservation about support groups, especially for PTSD sufferers, is that they can encourage dwelling on the past and actually prevent people from making necessary changes in their lives. Groups that help anxious people address the source of their anxieties and change maladaptive ways of thinking and behaving are most effective.

## SPIRITUAL PRACTICE

A regular spiritual practice can provide structure and solace in late life. Such a connection seems to offer tangible benefits and a sense of hope that can aid seniors in coping with the multiple issues of aging.

In a study I conducted on how people coped with Alzheimer's and cancer, we found that the strongest predictors of emotional strength weren't how sick family members were or how much money they had, but the strength of their spiritual beliefs.[9] In this study, what affected their coping wasn't the frequency with which people attended formal church services but the inner strength and support they garnered from their beliefs.

Other research funded by the National Institute of Aging indicates that seniors who were involved in religious activities had higher levels of well-being, less depression and cognitive difficulties, and a four-time lower suicide rate than the general population.[10] Visits with friends or family did not correlate with reduced suicide rates, so the protective effect was not a result of social contact but rather, according to the authors, of "a unique role that religious involvement could contribute to preventing suicide."

The elderly who participated in religious services showed improved emotional well-being, including increased optimism and less depressive symptoms. They also had stronger support systems and social ties and a lower frequency of unhealthy behaviors.

This has been borne out by many of my patients, including Detoh, a ninety-five-year-old nursing home resident who reflected on the importance of religion in her life.

"This is the stage in my life when my faith means the most," she told me. "So much of what used to be vital has passed away—my husband, most of my friends, my hearing—but I can hold on to this. I get comfort in the thought of an afterlife and that my life has meant something. I don't go to church much anymore, but I'd say my faith is stronger than ever."

## VOLUNTEERING

Volunteering can be an especially powerful activity for the elderly, providing needed structure and instilling a sense of accomplishment and pride.

Research indicates that older people who volunteer gain numerous mental-health benefits. Programs like the mentoring program Nancy's father joined allow seniors to utilize their life experiences and skills. There are numerous programs that recruit and train retired professionals, such as doctors, lawyers, and accountants, to counsel and advise in the community, but volunteering for a local school, scout troop, or recreation center can be just as beneficial.

AOA, the Administration on Aging in the U.S. Department of Health and Human Services, is composed of a web of agencies that rely on older Americans to volunteer in a wide range of areas.

The Senior Corps, the federal agency for senior volunteers, offers a number of programs, including the Foster Grandparents Program, where volunteers give support to special-needs children; the Senior Companion Program, where volunteers help other elderly maintain their independence; and Family Friends, a program that matches older adults with at-risk children and families.

Other options include community and faith-based programs such as literary programs, meal delivery, and visits to homebound seniors. These activities can give those in late life a sense of purpose, as well as providing the community with the benefits of their wisdom and skills.

"When I retired I felt useless, like my life was over," a depressed patient named Lawrence told me. "I'd been a social worker all my life, and I still had a lot of knowledge and caring left in me. My granddaughter convinced me that I'd feel better if I stayed involved with helping others, and she was so right. I'm energized by my volunteer work with other seniors who are trying to remain independent at home."

## NUTRITION ISSUES

**Changes in eating habits.** Anxious seniors, especially those living alone, often eat erratically or snack on junk food that is full of empty calories rather than having regular nutritious meals. The ramifications of a poor diet in late life can be dramatic, affecting brain function and causing dehydration that leads to disorientation and confusion.

On a visit to her out-of-town mother, Lucille found that she had been subsisting almost entirely on ice cream and cookies, despite the fact that Lucille had ordered a weekly grocery delivery. "The refrigerator was full of items she would have once used to make her dinner, but she had become too overwhelmed to put them together. I hadn't realized this till I visited her. So I did a little investigating and ended up signing her up for Meals on Wheels."

Meals on Wheels charges a modest amount for a one- or two-meal-a-day home delivery service, and also prepares foods for special diets. Another inexpensive and convenient option is a local senior center that provides a daily meal, along with recreational services, encouraging an anxious parent to socialize as well as eat at least one meal a day.

Researchers at the Tufts University Center on Nutrition modified the

USDA's food guide pyramid for seniors over seventy. Since dehydration is often a problem for older people, resulting in kidney problems and constipation, a major modification is the inclusion of eight or more glasses of water per day. Another modification is the addition of extra fiber, which is especially essential for digestion in late life.[11]

**Vitamin deficiencies.** Tuft researchers also suggested the addition of calcium, vitamin D, and vitamin B-12 supplements to senior diets. B vitamins are essential for balanced mood and brain functioning. Deficiencies in these vitamins, which can be a result of poor eating habits, are often linked with depression.

**Caffeine intake.** Caffeine is a stimulant that can interfere with sleep and cause or exacerbate anxiety symptoms, increasing feelings of panic and restlessness. Caffeine is present not only in tea and coffee, but also in many sodas, chocolate, and some over-the-counter headache remedies, such as Excedrin. Eliminating caffeine from the diet or reducing it to a minimum can dramatically reduce anxiety and nervousness.

Diet products that contain stimulants such as ephedra also have stimulant properties and can cause anxiety symptoms.

**Sugar and hypoglycemia.** The symptoms of hypoglycemia, a below-normal level of blood sugar, are the same as for many anxiety disorders—lightheadedness, palpitations, nervousness, weakness, sweating, and a feeling of panic. If low blood sugar is a problem, eating smaller, protein-based meals or snacks four or five times a day, along with less white sugar and starches, can be beneficial.

**Alcohol.** Often used to counteract stress, alcohol is actually a depressant that can suppress dreaming sleep, trigger anxiety, and increase depression. Because of this, alcohol use should be minimized in the anxious elderly, especially those with other physical ailments.

**Omega-3 fatty acids.** Some experts believe that depression is linked to a deficiency of these substances, which are plentiful in fish and nuts. Some research has shown that patients who were unresponsive to standard antidepressants found that a daily dose of omega-3 fatty acid resulted in a decrease in symptoms such as anxiety, sadness, and sleeping difficulties. Since there is also evidence that omega-3s may help alleviate arthritis and help prevent heart disease, adding fish, nuts, or flaxseed to the diet, or a fish-oil supplement such as eicosapentaenoic acid (EPA), may be beneficial.

**Nicotine** is not only addictive, but a stimulant as well. It can cause agitation and contribute to general anxiety and ill health. Most people need to withdraw slowly from nicotine, and medications are now available to help decrease the craving for it.

# THE COMFORT OF PETS

I know an elderly woman, legally blind, who lives alone with her golden retriever. Many mornings on my way to work, I see her with her cane in one hand and a leash in the other, walking along the lane that borders her house.

"How does she manage on her own?" I once asked a niece who was visiting her.

"It's her dog," she told me. "She was so distraught and depressed when she began losing her sight. She got her dog as a seeing-eye helper, but he ended up helping her cope just as much with her loneliness and panic."

Research reinforces the fact that having a pet can positively affect an elderly person's mental physical health. One study reported that independently living seniors with pets, for instance a dog or a cat, tended to have better mental well-being and physical health than non–pet owners. They coped better with stress, remained more active, and were better equipped to remain emotionally stable during crises.[12]

## HOW HAVING A PET CAN HELP IN LATE LIFE

**Combats loneliness.** Many seniors with anxiety disorders are isolated and bored. Handling and owning a pet is a way of providing companionship.

**Gives purpose.** Taking care of a pet can provide a sense of purposefulness to an anxious parent, whose days otherwise might be open-ended and without meaning. A pet requires daily feeding, watering, grooming, and walking, which can establish a much-needed routine and schedule.

**Provides physical contact.** Studies suggest that the physical contact of petting an animal is relaxing and can improve mood and even lower blood pressure. For anxious parents who live far from family and friends, touching an animal may be the only regular physical contact they have.

**Encourages exercise and interaction.** Walking a dog—or even a cat—can provide an anxious elderly person with daily exercise, a chance to be outdoors, and a way to have contact with other pet owners. For the isolated anxious, who have difficulty leaving the house, this can be particularly beneficial.

**Provides unconditional love.** Seniors often find a much-needed source of love and comfort from a pet during a time of life when loss of spouses and friends is common.

## Considering a Pet

**Living quarters.** Dogs and cats may not be allowed in apartments and retirement communities. In these cases, a caged bird, guinea pig, or even an aquarium could provide some of the benefits.

**Match the person and pet.** The physical condition of an anxious parent is important to consider. A puppy may be too harrowing for an elderly person to train, while an older, house-trained dog might be a better option. Cats are a good option for those who are more frail and cannot handle daily walks.

**Find a pet-friendly environment.** Many nursing homes and assisted-living facilities encourage pet visitors. I am often amazed when I see a very withdrawn person come alive when a dog or cat is brought in for a visit. Eden Alternative, a network of residential homes for seniors, allows dogs, birds, and cats, and includes an outside environment with farm animals such as rabbits and chickens.

**Try pet services.** For those living in nursing homes or retirement homes, services such as Pets on Wheels and Therapy Dogs International bring pets to assisted-living homes and hospitals so that the elderly can interact with them.

**Let your parent decide.** Even though it may seem that a pet is a good idea for a parent, owning a pet is a serious, long-term commitment, and a decision that your parent alone should make.

# SLEEP

Anyone who suffers from high stress and anxiety has tales of sleepless nights spent lying awake with a churning mind and a restless body. We don't need medical research to tell us lack of sleep leaves us diminished and frazzled.

Anxiety and stress have a direct effect on sleep. A lack of sound sleep is linked to excess levels of cortisol, the hormone that triggers stress. One of the many reasons why sleep is so important is that it gives the body respite from the chronic production of these hormones. When we sleep deeply, our bodies are receiving a much-needed break.

Lack of exercise, excessive caffeine or nicotine, and late-night TV watching have all been implicated in sleep difficulties. Insomnia can also be a side effect of a number of antidepressants, including SSRIs, though this effect often diminishes with time.

If insomnia is a chronic problem, relaxation techniques or medication may be helpful. Daytime exercise can help improve nighttime sleeping. I occasionally prescribe Ambien to help patients sleep, but it should not be taken every night. Over-the-counter alternatives such as melatonin have shown some effectiveness, but they should only be taken under the supervision of a physician, because they can have side effects.

# DON'T FORGET LAUGHTER

Bill Cosby said, "If you can laugh at it, you can survive it."

There may be no quicker fix for a bout of anxiety or sadness than a good dose of humor. When we laugh, our muscles relax, our blood pressure is reduced, and endorphins are released. Laughter can help reduce tension even in very difficult situations. For example, I encourage caregivers of people with dementia to laugh if something humorous happens, and to realize that they are laughing *with*—not *at*—the ill person.

Humor is a uniting force that cuts across status, sex, cultures, and age groups. It costs nothing, and can be given freely to friends and strangers alike. Humor provides perspective and allows us to step out of ourselves and see the irony and insignificance of seemingly unsolvable problems.

We know that humor and laughter make us feel better, but now there is scientific evidence that it's physically beneficial. Studies have suggested that laughter has a positive effect on immunity, and counterbalances the dangerous effects of stress by lowering the levels of cortisol, which adrenal glands secrete during tense times. To tune into the healing qualities of laughter:

- Watch a funny video
- Share jokes with a friend
- Read a humorous book
- Look for funny anecdotes in newspapers
- Encourage playfulness

You might even try to force a laugh. Exaggerate your situation out of proportion until it becomes ridiculous—then laugh at it.

## QUICK ANXIETY FIXES

Another way to quickly banish anxiety is to become involved in a pleasurable activity that provides a shift of focus and a distraction from worry or fear.

- Listen to classical music
- Read poetry out loud or memorize a short poem
- Read an inspirational book
- Listen to an audiobook
- Sing
- Call or visit a friend
- Take a brisk walk
- Garden
- Do a crossword puzzle
- Arrange a bouquet of flowers
- Walk your dog, or visit a friend's
- Help someone else
- Watch a video of a favorite comedy
- Play with a child
- Give and take love and affection—wherever you can

The human requirement for love may actually be a physical necessity, as vital to us as certain nutrients and vitamins in keeping our brains functioning properly.

We know—even without studies—that there may be no more therapeutic ally than love. Love and support from friends and relatives are often the best anxiety treatments of all.

# NOTES

## CHAPTER 1

1. The Mellman Group conducted a telephone survey of 500 residents, living on or south of Canal Street, May 2–6, 2002.
2. Susan Gilbert, "For Depression, the Family Doctor May Be the First Choice but Not the Best," *The New York Times,* June 24, 2003.
3. M. Hamilton, "The Assessment of Anxiety States by Rating," *Br J Med Psychol* 32 (1959) :50–59.

## CHAPTER 2

1. Ian Smith, "Brain Scan Can Predict Response to Antidepressant," *Neuropsychopharmacology,* July 2003.
2. Greg Easterbrook, *The Progress Paradox* (New York: Random House, 2003), p. 194.
3. Jerome Groopman, *The Anatomy of Hope* (New York: Random House, 2003).
4. I. Kaplan, Benjamin Sadock, and Jack Grebb, *Synopsis of Psychiatry, Behavioral Sciences, Clinical Psychiatry* (Baltimore: Williams & Wilkins, 1991).

5. "Fear in the Amygdala," Health Agencies Update, *JAMA* 288, no. 7 (August 21, 2002).

6. George Zubenko et al., "Genome-wide linkage survey for genetic loci that influence the development of depressive disorders in families with recurrent, early-onset major depression," *American Journal of Medical Genetics,* Part B: *Neuropsychiatric Genetics,* July 2003.

7. Jerome Groopman, *The Anatomy of Hope* (New York: Random House, 2003).

## CHAPTER 3

1. S. M. Neikrug, "Worrying about a Frightening Old Age," *Aging & Mental Health* 7, no. 5 (September 2003):326–333.

## CHAPTER 4

1. J. J. Gallo, W. Reichel, and L. Andersen, *Handbook of Geriatric Assessment,* 3rd ed. (Gaithersburg, MD: Aspen Publishers, 2000).

2. George Zubenko et al., "Genome-wide linkage survey for genetic loci that influence the development of depressive disorders in families with recurrent, early-onset major depression," *American Journal of Medical Genetics,* Part B: *Neuropsychiatric Genetics,* July 2003.

3. Golden et al., "A Longitudinal Study of Serotonergic Function in Depression," *Neuropsychopharmacology* 26 (2002):653–659.

4. T. L. Brink, J. A. Yesavage, O. Lum, P. Heersema, M. B. Adey, and T. L. Rose, "Screening tests for geriatric depression," *Clinical Gerontologist* 1 (1982): 37–44.

5. J. A. Yesavage et al., "Development and validation of a geriatric depression screening scale: A preliminary report," *Journal of Psychiatric Research* 17 (1983):37–49.

CHAPTER 5

1. E. H. Uhlenhuth, M. B. Balter, G. D. Mellinger, I. H. Cisin, and J. Clinthorne, "Symptom checklist syndromes in the general population: correlations with psychotherapeutic drug use," *Archives of General Psychiatry* 49 (1983):1167–1173.
2. Edmund J. Bourne, *The Anxiety & Phobia Workbook* (Oakland, CA: New Harbinger Publications, 1995).
3. "Fear in the Amygdala," Health Agencies Update, *JAMA* 288, no. 7 (August 21, 2002).
4. Harold Kaplan, Benjamin Sacock, and Jack Grebb, *A Synopsis of Psychiatry* (Baltimore: Williams & Wilkins, 1995).

CHAPTER 6

1. L. N. Robins and D. Regier, eds., *Psychiatric Disorders in America* (New York: Free Press, 1991).
2. Harold Kaplan, Benjamin Sacock, and Jack Grebb, *A Synopsis of Psychiatry* (Baltimore: Williams & Wilkins, 1995).
3. Michele T. Pato, *Best Practice of Medicine,* November 2000, Professional Reference. Merck Medicus, http://merck.praxis.md/index.
4. Edmund J. Bourne, *The Anxiety & Phobia Workbook* (Oakland, CA: New Harbinger Publications, 1995).

CHAPTER 7

1. C. S. North, S. I. Nixon, S. Shariat, S. Mallonee, J. C. McMillen, E. L. Spitznagel, and E. M. Smith, "Psychiatric disorders among survivors of the Oklahoma City bombing," *JAMA* 282 (August 25, 1999):755–762.
2. Ben Shepperd, *A War of Nerves* (Cambridge, MA: Harvard, 2000).
3. M. Stein et al., "Genetic and Environmental Influences on Trauma Exposure

and Posttraumatic Stress Disorder Symptoms: A Twin Study," *Am J Psychiatry* 159 (2002):1675–1681.

4. J. H. Shore, "Psychiatric reactions to disaster: The Mount St. Helens experience," *Am J Psychiatry* 143 (1986):590–595.

5. R. L. Swank, "Combat Exhaustion," *Journal of Nervous and Mental Diseases* 109 (1949):475–506.

6. Jerome Groopman, *The Anatomy of Hope* (New York: Random House, 2003).

7. F. Donata et al., "Cognitive Behavioral Therapy and Aerobic Exercise for Gulf War Veterans' Illnesses: A Randomized Controlled Trial," *JAMA* 289 (March 19, 2003):1396–1403.

8. David Berreby, "War's Psychic Toll, From Homer On," *The New York Times* large-type weekly, March 17–23, 2003.

## Chapter 8

1. L. N. Robins and D. Regier, eds., *Psychiatric Disorders in America* (New York: Free Press, 1991).

2. Harold Kaplan, Benjamin Sacock, and Jack Grebb, *A Synopsis of Psychiatry* (Baltimore: Williams & Wilkins, 1995).

3. Anahad O'Connor, "Panic Spells Are Traced to Chemical in the Brain," *The New York Times,* January 27, 2004.

4. Guillern Massana et al., "Parahippocampal Gray Matter Density in Panic Disorder, a Voxel-Based Morphometric Study," *Am J Psychiatry* 160 (March 2003):3.

## Chapter 9

1. M. Manela, C. Katona, and G. Livingston, "How common are the anxiety disorders in old age?" *International Journal of Geriatric Psychiatry* 11 (1996):65–70.

2. S. Mannuzza, F. R. Schneier, T. F. Chapman, M. R. Liebowitz, D. F. Klein, and A. J. Fryer, "Generalized social phobia reliability and validity," *Arch Gen Psychiatry* 52 (1995):23–37.

3. Jerome Kagan, *The Nature of the Child* (New York: Basic Books, 1994).

4. Eric Hollander and Dan J. Stein, eds., *Textbook of Anxiety Disorders* (Washington, DC: American Psychiatric Publishing, 2002).

5. Murray B. Stein et al., "Increased Amygdala Activation to Angry and Contemptuous Faces in Generalized Social Phobia," *Arch Gen Psychiatry* 59 (2002): 1027–1034.

6. Yadin Dudai, "Fear Thou Not," *Nature* 421 (January 2003).

## CHAPTER 10

1. Geoffrey Cowley, "Our Bodies, Our Fears," *Newsweek*, February 24, 2003.

2. Greg Miller, "Pills and games help conquer fear," *Science* 302 (November 2003).

## CHAPTER 11

1. Roger J. Cadieux, "Antidepressant drug interaction in the elderly," *Postgraduate Medicine* 106, 6 (November 1999).

2. *The New York Times,* Large Type Weekly, March 17–23, 2003.

3. J. R. Mort and R. R. Aparasu, "Prescribing potentially inappropriate psychotropic medications to the ambulatory elderly," *Archives of Internal Medicine* 160 (2000):2825–2831.

4. Erica Goode, "Leading Drugs for Psychosis Come Under New Scrutiny," *The New York Times,* May 20, 2003.

5. B. M. Cohen et al., "Effects of the novel antidepressant S-adenosylmethionine on alpha-1 and beta-adrenoreceptors on brain," *Eur J Pharmacol* 170 (1989): 201–207.

## CHAPTER 12

1. F. Li, P. Harmer, E. McAuley, et al., "An evaluation of tai chi exercise on physical function among older persons: A randomized controlled trial," *Annals of Behavioral Medicine* 23 (2001):139–146.

2. C. H. Patel, "Yoga and bio-feedback in the management of hypertension," *Lancet* 2 (1973):1973–1975.

3. Richard Davidson et al., "Alterations in Brain and Immune Function Produced by Mindfulness Meditation," *Psychosomatic Medicine* 65 (2003):564–570.

4. Kimberly Williams, "Mindfulness training program and yoga," West Virginia University, Morgantown, *American Journal of Health Promotion,* July 2001.

5. G. Greendale, "Yoga for Women With Hyperkyphosis: Results of a Pilot Study," *American Journal of Public Health* 92 (2002):1611–1614.

6. Martin Seligman, *Learned Optimism: How to Change Your Mind and Your Life* (New York: Free Press, 1998).

7. Greg Easterbrook. *The Progress Paradox* (New York: Random House, 2004).

## CHAPTER 13

1. Greg Easterbrook, *The Progress Paradox* (New York: Random House, 2004).

2. Paul Wiseman, "Okinawan Seniors Aren't as Lonely," USAToday.com, April 2003.

3. Walter Bortz. *Dare to Be 100* (New York: Simon & Schuster, 1996).

4. S. J. H. Biddle and N. Mutrie, *Psychology of Physical Activity and Exercise* (London: Springer Verlag, 1991).

5. Andrew Well, *Spontaneous Healing* (New York: Fawcett Columbine, 1995), p. 188.

6. D. Spiegel, "Healing Words: Emotional Expression and Disease Outcome," *Journal of the American Medical Association* 280 (1999):1328–1329.

7. J. M. Smyth, A. A. Stone, A. Hurewitz, and A. Kaell, "Effects of Writing about Stressful Experiences on Symptom Reduction in Patients with Asthma or Rheumatoid Arthritis: A Randomized Trial," *Journal of the American Medical Association* 281 (1999):1304–1309.

8. L. Teri, R. Logsdon, J. Uomoto, and S. M. McCurry, "Behavioral treatment of depression in dementia patients: A controlled clinical trial," *Journal of Gerontology: Psychological Sciences* 52B (1997):159–166.

9. P. V. Rabins, M. D. Fitting, J. Eastham, and J. Zabora, "Emotional adaptation

over time in caregivers for the chronically ill elderly," *Age and Ageing* 19 (1990):185–190.

10. Peter Van Ness and David Larson, "Religion, senescence, and mental health: The end of life is not the end of hope," *American Journal of Geriatric Psychiatry* 10 (2002):386–397.

11. Tufts University Center on Nutrition, online at www.Navigator.tufts.edu.

12. P. Raina, D. Waltner-Toews, B. Bonnett, et al., "Influence of companion animals on the physical and psychological health of older people: An analysis of a one-year longitudinal study," *Journal of the American Geriatrics Society* 47 (March 1999):323–329.

# BIBLIOGRAPHY

## CAREGIVING

Anderson, Ellis, and Marsha Dryan. *Aging Parents & You.* New York: Master Media Limited, 1988.

Berman, Claire. *Caring for Yourself While Caring for Your Aging Parents.* New York: Henry Holt, 2000.

Butler, Robert. *Why Survive? Being Old in America.* New York: Harper & Row, 1975.

Carter, Rosalynn. *Helping Yourself Help Others.* New York: Times Books, 1995.

Deane, Barbara. *Caring for Your Aging Parents: When Love Is Not Enough.* Colorado Springs, CO: Navpress, 1989.

Greenberg, Vivian. *Children of a Certain Age: Adults and Their Aging Parents.* New York: Macmillan, 1994.

Greenberg, Vivian. *Respecting Your Limits When Caring for Aging Parents.* Somerset, NJ: Jossey-Bass, 1998.

Greenberg, Vivian. *Your Best Is Good Enough: Aging Parents and Your Emotions.* New York: Lexington Books, 1989.

Halpern, James. *Helping Your Aging Parents: A Practical Guide for Adult Children.* New York: Fawcett Crest, 1987.

Heath, Angela. *Long-Distance Caregiving*. Lakewood, CO: American Source Books, 1993.

Jarvik, Lissy, and Garry Small. *Parentcare: A Commonsense Guide for Adult Children*. New York: Crown Publishers, 1988.

La Buda, Dennis R., and Vicki Schmall. *Home Sweet Home: How to Help Older Adults Live Independently*. Appleton, WI: Quality Life Resources, 2000.

Lebow, Grace, et al. *Coping with Your Difficult Older Parent: A Guide for Stressed-Out Children*. New York: HarperCollins, 1999.

Levin, Norma Jean. *How to Care for Your Parents: A Practical Guide to Eldercare*. New York: W. W. Norton, 1997.

Llardo, Joseph A. *As Parents Age*. Acton, MA: VanderWyk & Burnham, 1998.

Mace, Nancy L., and Peter V. Rabins. *The 36-Hour Day: A Family Guide to Caring for Persons with Alzheimer's Disease, Related Dementing Illnesses, and Memory Loss in Later Life*. Baltimore: Johns Hopkins University Press, 1999.

Marcell, Jacqueline. *Elder Rage, or Take My Father . . . Please! How to Survive Caring for Aging Parents*. Irvine, CA: Impressive Press, 2001.

McLeod, Beth W. *Caregiving: The Spiritual Journey of Love, Loss and Renewal*. New York: John Wiley & Sons, 1999.

Morris, V. Butler. *How to Care for Aging Parents*. New York: Workman Press, 1996.

Myers, Edward. *When Parents Die*. New York: Penguin, 1997.

Nuland, Sherwin B. *How We Die*. New York: Alfred A. Knopf, 1994.

Pritkin, Enid, and Trudy Reece. *Parentcare Survival Guide*. Hauppauge, NY: Barron's, 1993.

Rhodes, Linda Colvin. *Complete Idiot's Guide to Caring for Aging Parents*. New York: Alpha Books, 2001.

Rob, Caroline. *The Caregiver's Guide*. New York: Houghton Mifflin, 1991.

Secunda, Victoria. *Losing Your Parent*. New York: Hyperion, 2000.

Silverstone, Barbara, and Helen Kandel Hyman. *You and Your Aging Parent*. New York: Pantheon, 1989.

Strauss, Peter, and Nancy Lederman. *The Elder Law Handbook: A Legal and Financial Survival Guide for Caregivers and Seniors*. New York: Facts on File, 1996.

## CREATIVITY

Cameron, Julia. *The Artist's Way: A Spiritual Path to Higher Creativity*. New York: Jeremy P. Tarcher, 1992.

Goldberg, Natalie. *Writing Down the Bones: Freeing the Writer Within*. Boston: Shambhala Publications, 1986.

Lamott, Anne. *Bird by Bird: Some Instructions on Writing and Life*. New York: Doubleday, 1994.

Lauber, Lynn. *Listen to Me: Writing Life into Meaning*. New York: Norton, 2003.

Polking, Kirk. *Writing Family Histories and Memoirs*. Cincinnati: Betterway Books, 1995.

Thomas, Frank P. *How to Write the Story of Your Life*. Cincinnati: Writers Digest Books, 1993.

Zimmerman, Susan. *Writing to Heal the Soul: Transforming Grief and Loss Through Writing*. New York: Three Rivers Press, 2001.

## DEPRESSION

Burns, D. D. *The Feeling Good Handbook*, rev. ed. New York: Plume, 1999.

Copeland, M. E. *The Depression Workbook: A Guide for Living with Depression*. Oakland, CA: New Harbinger Publications, 2000.

Jamison, Kay Redfield. *An Unquiet Mind*. New York: Random House, 1997.

Klein, D. F., and P. H. Wender. *Do You Have a Depressive Illness? How to Tell, What to Do*. New York: HarperCollins, 1990.

Klein, Donald F., and Anne Sheffield. *How You Can Survive When They're Depressed: Living and Coping with Depression Fallout*. New York: Crown, 1999.

Lovestone, Simon. *Depression in Elderly People*. London: Martin Dunitz, 1996.

Luciani, Joseph J. *Self-Coaching: How to Heal Anxiety and Depression*. New York: John Wiley & Sons, 2001.

Real, Terrence. *I Don't Want to Talk About It: Overcoming the Secret Legacy of Male Depression*. New York: Scribner, 1998.

Rosen, Laura Epstein, and Xavier F. Amador. *When Someone You Love Is De-*

*pressed: How to Help Your Loved One Without Losing Yourself.* New York: Free Press, 1997.

Yapko, Michael D. *Hand-Me-Down Blues: How to Stop Depression from Spreading in Families.* New York: Griffin, 2000.


## GENERALIZED ANXIETY DISORDER

Bourne, E. J. *The Anxiety and Phobia Workbook.* Oakland, CA: New Harbinger Publications, 1995.

Butler, G., and T. Hope. *Managing Your Mind: The Mental Fitness Game.* New York: Oxford University Press, 1995.

Copeland, Mary Ellen. *The Worry Control Workbook.* Oakland, CA: New Harbinger Publications, 1998.

Eshelman, Davis M., and M. McKay. *The Relaxation and Stress Reduction Workbook,* 5th ed. Oakland, CA: New Harbinger Publications, 1995.


## HUMOR

Blumenfeld, E., and L. Alpern. *Humor at Work.* Atlanta: Peachtree Publishers, 1994.

Cousins, Norman. *Anatomy of an Illness as Perceived by the Patient.* New York: W. W. Norton, 1979.

Klein, Allen. *Healing Power of Humor.* Los Angeles: Tarcher, 1989.

Kushner, Malcolm. *The Light Touch.* New York: Simon & Schuster, 1990.

McGhee, Paul. *Health, Healing and the Amuse System.* Dubuque, IA: Kendall/Hunt, 1996.

Morreall, John. *Humor Works.* Amherst, MA: HRD Press, 1997.

Paulson, Terry. *Making Humor Work.* Los Altos, CA: Crisp Publishing, 1989.

Robinson, Vera. *Humor and the Health Professions,* 2nd ed. Thorofare, NJ: Charles B. Slack, 1991.

Weinstein, Matt. *Managing to Have Fun.* New York: Simon & Schuster, 1997.

## Medication

Albers, Lawrence J., M.D. *Handbook of Psychiatric Drugs*. 2004 ed. New York: Current Clinical Strategies, 2003.

Appleton, William S. *Prozac and the New Antidepressants: What You Need to Know*. New York: Plume, 2000.

Drummond, Edward. *The Complete Guide to Psychiatric Drugs: Straight Talk for Best Results*. New York: John Wiley & Sons, 2000.

Gorman, Jack. *The Essential Guide to Psychiatric Drugs*. New York: St. Martin's Press, 1992.

Graedon, Teresa, and Joe Graedon. *Deadly Drug Interactions: The People's Pharmacy Guide*. New York: St. Martin's Press, 1999.

Kramer, Peter F. *Listening to Prozac*. New York: Penguin, 1997.

Lininger, S., ed. *The A–Z Guide to Drug-Herb and Vitamin Interactions*. Rocklin, CA: Prima, 1999.

Lininger, S., A. Gaby, and J. Miller, eds. *The Natural Pharmacy*. Rocklin, CA: Prima, 1999.

Opler, Lewis A., and Carol Bialkowski. *Prozac and Other Psychiatric Drugs*. New York: Pocket Books, 1996.

Rybacki, James J., and James W. Long. *The Essential Guide to Prescription Drugs 2004: Everything You Need to Know for Safe Drug Use*. New York: Hyper-Resource, 2003.

Turkington, Carol Ann, and Eliot F. Kaplan. *Making the Prozac Decision: A Guide to Antidepressants*. Los Angeles: Lowell House, 1994.

## Obsessive-compulsive Disorder

Baer, L. *Getting Control: Overcoming Your Obsessions and Compulsions,* rev. ed. New York: Plume, 2000.

de Silva, P., and S. J. Rachman. *Obsessive-Compulsive Disorder: The Facts,* 2nd ed. New York: Oxford University Press, 1998.

Fineberg, Naomi, ed. *Obsessive-Compulsive Disorder: A Practical Guide*. London: Taylor & Francis, 2001.

Foa, E. B., and M. J. Kozak. *Mastery of Your Obsessive-Compulsive Disorder* (client workbook). San Antonio, TX: The Psychological Corporation, 1997.

Foa, E. B., and R. Wilson. *Stop Obsessing! How to Overcome Your Obsessions and Compulsions,* rev. ed. New York: Bantam, 2001.

Gravitz, H. L. *Obsessive-Compulsive Disorder: New Help for the Family.* Santa Barbara, CA: Healing Visions Press, 1998.

Hyman, B. M., and C. Pedrick. *The OCD Workbook: Your Guide to Breaking Free From Obsessive-Compulsive Disorder.* Oakland, CA: New Harbinger Publications, 1999.

Jenike, M. A., L. Baer, and W. E. Minichiello, eds. *Obsessive-Compulsive Disorders: Practical Management,* 2nd ed. New York: Mosby, 1988.

Neziroglu, F. A., and J. A. Yaryura-Tobias. *Over and Over Again: Understanding Obsessive-Compulsive Behavior.* Lexington, MA: D. C. Heath, 1991.

Penzel, F. *Obsessive-Compulsive Disorders: Getting Well and Staying Well.* New York: Oxford University Press, 2000.

Rapoport, J. L. *The Boy Who Couldn't Stop Washing—The Experience and Treatment of Obsessive-Compulsive Disorder.* New York: New American Library, 1989.

Ross, Jerilyn. *Triumph Over Fear.* New York: Bantam Books, 1994.

Schwartz, J. M. *Brain Lock: Free Yourself from Obsessive-Compulsive Behavior.* New York: Regan Books, 1996.

Steketee, G. S. *Overcoming Obsessive-Compulsive Disorder* (client manual). Oakland, CA: New Harbinger Publications, 1999.

Steketee, G., and K. White. *When Once Is Not Enough: Help for Obsessive-Compulsives.* Oakland, CA: New Harbinger Publications, 1990.

Summers, M. *Everything in Its Place: My Trials and Triumphs with Obsessive-Compulsive Disorder.* New York: Jeremy P. Tarcher, 1999.

## PANIC DISORDER

Clum, George A. *Coping with Panic: A Drug-Free Approach to Dealing with Anxiety Attacks.* Pacific Grove, CA: Brooks/Cole, 1990.

Craske, M. G., and D. H. Barlow. *Mastery of Your Anxiety and Panic,* 3rd ed. (MAP-3). San Antonio, TX: The Psychological Corporation, 2000.

Eldridge, G. D., and J. R. Walker. *Coping with Panic Workbook*. Blacksburg, VA: Self-Change Systems, 2000.

*Panic Disorder and Agoraphobia: A Guide*. Madison, WI: Obsessive-Compulsive Information Center, Madison Institute of Medicine, 2001.

Peurifoy, R. Z. *Anxiety, Phobias, and Panic: Taking Charge and Conquering Fear,* 2nd ed. Citrus Heights, CA: Lifeskills, 1992.

Rachman, S. J., and P. de Silva. *Panic Disorder: The Facts*. New York: Oxford University Press, 1996.

Wilson, R. R. *Breaking the Panic Cycle: Self-Help for People with Phobias*. Washington, DC: Anxiety Disorders Association of America, 1987.

Wilson, R. R. *Don't Panic: Taking Control of Anxiety Attacks*. New York: Harper & Row, 1996.

Znercher-White, E. *An End to Panic: Breakthrough Techniques for Overcoming Panic Disorder,* 2nd ed. Oakland, CA: New Harbinger Publications, 1997.

## PHOBIA (SOCIAL)

Antony, M. M., and R. P. Swinson. *The Shyness and Social Anxiety Workbook: Proven, Step-by-Step Techniques for Overcoming Your Fear*. Oakland, CA: New Harbinger Publications, 2000.

Beidel, D. C., and S. Turner. *Shy Children, Phobic Adults: Nature and Treatment of Social Phobia*. Washington, DC: American Psychological Association, 1997.

Bower, S. A., and G. H. Bower. *Asserting Yourself.* Menlo Park, CA: Addison-Wesley, 1965.

Carducci, B. J. *Shyness: A Bold New Approach. The Latest Scientific Findings, Plus Practical Steps for Finding Your Comfort Zone*. New York: HarperCollins, 1999.

Carmin, C. N., C. A. Pollard, T. Flynn, and B. G. Markway. *Dying of Embarrassment: Help for Social Anxiety and Phobia*. Oakland, CA: New Harbinger Publications, 1992.

Cheek, J. M. *Conquering Shyness*. New York: Basic Books, 1990.

Hope, D. A., R. G. Heimberg, H. R. Juster, and C. L. Turk. *Managing Social Anxiety*. San Antonio, TX: The Psychological Corporation, 2000.

Johnson, D. W. *Reaching Out, Interpersonal Effectiveness and Self-Actualization.* Englewood Cliffs, NJ: Prentice-Hall, 1999.

Leary, M. R., and R. M. Kowalski. *Social Anxiety.* New York: Guilford Press, 1995.

Markway, B. G., and G. P. Markway. *Painfully Shy: How to Overcome Social Anxiety and Reclaim Your Life.* New York: Thomas Dunne Books, St. Martin's Press, 2001.

Marshall, J. *Social Phobia: From Shyness to Stage Fright.* New York: Basic Books, 1995.

McKay, M., and P. Fanning. *Self-Esteem.* Oakland, CA: New Harbinger Publications, 1987.

Rapee, R. M. *Overcoming Shyness and Social Phobia: A Step-by-Step Guide.* Northvale, NJ: Jason Aronson, 1998.

Robin, M. W., and R. Balter. *Performance Anxiety: Overcoming Your Fear in the Workplace, Social Situations, Interpersonal Communications, the Performing Arts.* Holbrook, MA: Adams Media Corporation, 1994.

Schneier, F., and L. Welkowitz. *The Hidden Face of Shyness: Understanding and Overcoming Social Anxiety.* New York: Avon Books, 1996.

Smith, M. J. *When I Say No I Feel Guilty.* New York: Bantam Books, 1975.

Stein, Murray B., and John R. Walker. *Triumph Over Shyness. Conquering Shyness and Social Anxiety.* New York: McGraw-Hill, 2001.

Zimbardo, P. G. *Shyness: What It Is, What to Do About It.* Reading, MA: Addison-Wesley Publishers, 1997.

## PHOBIAS (SPECIFIC)

Antony, M. M., M. G. Craske, and D. H. Barlow. *Mastery of Your Specific Phobia* (client workbook). San Antonio, TX: The Psychological Corporation; Boulder, CO: Graywind Publications, 1995.

Bourne, E. J. *Overcoming Specific Phobia: A Hierarchy and Exposure-Based Protocol for the Treatment of All Specific Phobias* (client manual). Oakland, CA: New Harbinger Publications, 1998.

Brown, D. *Flying Without Fear.* Oakland, CA: New Harbinger Publications, 1996.

Hartman, C., and J. S. Huffaker. *The Fearless Flyer: How to Fly in Comfort and Without Trepidation.* Portland, OR: Eighth Mountain Press, 1995.

Zane, M. D., and H. Milt. *Your Phobia: Understanding Your Fears Through Contextual Therapy.* Washington, DC.: American Psychiatric Press, 1984.


## POSTTRAUMATIC STRESS DISORDER

Cohen, Barry M., Mary-Michola Barnes, and Anita B. Rankin. *Managing Traumatic Stress Through Art: Drawing From the Center.* Lutterville, MD: Sidran Press, 1995.

Matsakis, A. *I Can't Get Over It: A Handbook for Trauma Survivors,* 2nd ed. Oakland, CA: New Harbinger Publications, 1996.

Matsakis, A. *Survival Guilt: A Self-Help Guide.* Oakland, CA: New Harbinger Publications, 1999.

Matsakis, A. *Trust After Trauma: A Guide to Relationships for Survivors and Those Who Love Them.* Oakland, CA: New Harbinger Publications, 1998.

Rosenbloom, D., and M. B. Williams, with B. E. Watkins. *Life After Trauma: Workbook for Healing.* New York: The Guilford Press, 1999.

Staudacher, Carol. *Beyond Grief: A Guide for Recovering from the Death of a Loved One.* Oakland, CA: New Harbinger Publications, 1991.

Staudacher, Carol. *Men & Grief: A Guide for Men Surviving the Death of a Loved One, A Resource for Caregivers and Mental Health Professionals.* Oakland, CA: New Harbinger Publications, 1998.


## SPIRITUALITY

Dossey, Larry. *Recovering the Soul: A Scientific and Spiritual Search.* New York: Bantam, 1989.

Frankl, Viktor. *Man's Search for Meaning.* New York: Washington Square Press, 1998.

Moore, Thomas. *Care of the Soul: a Guide for Cultivating Depth and Sacredness in Everyday Life.* New York: HarperPerennial, 1994.

Peck, M. Scott. *The Road Less Traveled: A New Psychology of Love, Traditional Values and Spiritual Growth.* New York: Touchstone, 1978.

Zukav, Gary. *The Seat of the Soul.* New York: Fireside Books, 1990.


## TREATMENT

Antony, M. M., and R. P. Swinson. *When Perfect Isn't Good Enough: Strategies for Coping with Perfectionism.* Oakland, CA: New Harbinger Publications, 1998.

Barlow, David. *Anxiety and Its Disorders: The Nature and Treatment of Anxiety and Panic.* New York: Guilford Press, 1988.

Bourne, Edmund, and Lorna Garano. *Coping with Anxiety.* Oakland, CA: New Harbinger Publications, 2003.

Burns, David. *Feeling Good.* New York: Signet, 1981.

Carrington, Patricia. *Freedom in Meditation.* New York: Anchor Press, 1977.

Claiborn, J., and C. Pedrick. *The Habit Change Workbook: How to Break Bad Habits and Form Good Ones.* Oakland, CA: New Harbinger Publications, 2001.

Davidson, Jonathan. *The Anxiety Book: Developing Strength in the Face of Fear.* New York: Riverhead Books, 2003.

Davis, M., E. R. Eshelman, and M. McKay. *The Relaxation and Stress Reduction Workbook,* 4th ed. Oakland, CA: New Harbinger Publications, 1995.

Dupont, Robert, Elizabeth Spencer, and Caroline DuPont. *The Anxiety Cure: An Eight-Step Program for Getting Well.* New York: John Wiley & Sons, 1998.

Fanning, Patrick. *Visualization for Change.* Oakland, CA: New Harbinger Publications, 1988.

Fredericks, Carlton. *Psycho Nutrition.* New York: Grosset & Dunlap, 1976.

Gold, Mark S. *The Good News About Panic, Anxiety and Phobias.* New York: Villard Books, 1989.

Greenberger, D., and C. A. Padesky. *Mind Over Mood: Change How You Feel by Changing the Way You Think.* New York: Guilford Press, 1995.

Griest, J., James Jefferson, and Isaac Marks. *Anxiety and Its Treatment.* New York: Warner Books, 1986.

Groopman, Jerome. *The Anatomy of Hope: How Patients Prevail in the Face of Illness.* New York: Random House, 2003.

Hay, Louise. *You Can Heal Your Life.* Santa Monica, CA: Hay House, 1984.

Helmstetter, Shad. *The Self-Talk Solution.* New York: Pocket Books, 1987.

Helmstetter, Shad. *What to Say When You Talk to Yourself.* New York: Pocket Books, 1982.

Jacobsen, Edmund. *Progressive Relaxation.* Chicago: The University Press of Chicago, Midway Reprint, 1974.

Jampolsky, Gerald. *Good-Bye to Guilt.* New York: Bantam Books, 1985.

Jeffers, Susan. *Feel the Fear and Do It Anyway.* San Diego, CA: Harcourt, Brace, Jovanovich, 1987.

Luciani, J. *Self-Coaching: How to Heal Anxiety and Depression.* New York: John Wiley & Sons, 2001.

Mason, John. *Guide to Stress Reduction.* Berkeley, CA: Celestial Arts, 1985.

McKay, M., M. Davis, and P. Fanning. *Messages: The Communications Skills Book,* 2nd ed. Oakland, CA: New Harbinger Publications, 1995.

Neuman, Frederic. *Fighting Fear: The Eight-Week Program for Treating Your Own Phobia.* New York: Bantam Books, 1986.

Paterson, R. J. *The Assertiveness Workbook: How to Express Your Ideas and Stand Up for Yourself at Work and in Relationships.* Oakland, CA: New Harbinger Publications, 2000.

Peurifoy, Reneau. *Anxiety, Phobias & Panic: Taking Charge and Conquering Fear.* New York: Warner Books, 1985.

Seligman, Martin. *Authentic Happiness: Using the New Positive Psychology to Realize Your Potential for Lasting Fulfillment.* New York: Free Press, 2002.

Seligman, Martin. *Learned Optimism: How to Change Your Mind and Your Life.* New York: Free Press, 1998.

Silove, D., and V. Manicavasagar. *Overcoming Panic: A Self-Help Guide Using Cognitive Behavioural Techniques.* New York: New York University Press, 2001.

Weeks, C. *Hope and Help for Your Nerves.* New York: Hawthorne Books, 1969.

Weeks, C. *Peace From Nervous Suffering.* New York: Hawthorne Books, 1972.

Weil, Dr. Andrew. *Spontaneous Healing.* New York: Ballantine Books, 1995.

Wurtman, Judith. *Managing Your Mind and Mood Through Food.* New York: Perennial, 1988.

# RESOURCES

## Agoraphobia

ABIL, Inc. (Agoraphobics Building Independent Lives)
3805 Cutshaw Avenue, Suite 415
Richmond, VA 23230
(804) 353-3964
National network of support groups

Agoraphobics in Action, Inc.
P.O. Box 1662
Antioch, TN 37011
(615) 831-2383

A.I.M. (Agoraphobics in Motion)
1719 Crooks Street
Royal Oak, MI 48067-1306
(248) 547-0400
Twenty groups nationally

New Beginnings Foundation for Agoraphobia
P.O. Box 9327
Glendale, CA 91226
(818) 549-9966

## Alzheimer's

Alzheimer's Association
919 N. Michigan Avenue, Suite 1000
Chicago, IL 60611
(800) 272-3900
www.alz.org

## Caregiving

Administration on Aging
200 Independence Avenue, SW
Washington, DC 20201
(202) 401-4541
www.aoa.dhhs.gov
To locate the office on aging and nursing home ombudsmen in your locality.

Aging Network Services
440 East-West Highway, Suite 907
Bethesda, MD 20814
(301) 657-4329
www.agingnets.com
Nationwide network of private practice geriatric social workers who can serve
as care managers for older parents who live at a distance.

Aging Parents: The Family Survival Guide
Video series on caring for aging parents
www.agingparents.com
(888) 777-5585

Caregiver Survival Resources
Links; questions and answers about caregiving.
www.caregiver911.com

CaregiverZone
One-stop spot for caregiving information, services, and resources.
www.caregiverzone.com

Children of Aging Parents
1609 Woodbourne Road, Suite 302A
Levittown, PA 19057
(800) 227-7294

Family Caregiver Alliance
425 Bus Street, Suite 500
San Francisco, CA 94108
(800) 445-8106
Provides links, resource information and caregiving advice.
www.caregiver.org

National Alliance for Caregiving
Provides resource information and advice.
www.caregiving.org

National Association for Home Care
519 C Street, NE
Washington, DC 20002
(202) 547-7424

National Association of Professional Geriatric Care Managers
1604 North Country Club Road
Tucson, AZ 85716
(520) 881-8008
www.caremanager.org

National Family Caregiver Association
10605 Concord Street, Suite 501
Kensington, MD 20895
(800) 896-3650
www.nfcacares.org

National Federation Interfaith Caregivers Association
(816) 931-5442
www.NFIVC.org
Find local volunteers to help elderly parents.

## Depression

Depression Alliance Online
Message boards, information, and other online resources for people with depression.
www.depressionalliance.org

Depression/Suicide National Hopeline Network
1-800-SUICIDE
Provides access to trained telephone counselors 24 hours a day, 7 days a week.

Depressives.org
Support network.
www.depressives.org

DRADA
Depression and Related Disorders Association
www.drada.org

National Depressive and Manic Depressive Association
730 N. Franklin, Suite 501
Chicago, IL 60601
(312) 642-0049; (800) 826-3632
www.ndmda.org

National Foundation for Depressive Illness, Inc.
P.O. Box 2257
New York, NY 10016
(212) 268-4260; (800) 239-1265
www.depression.org

## MENTAL HEALTH ORGANIZATIONS

Alcoholics Anonymous
(212) 870-3400
www.alcoholics-anonymous.org

American Counseling Association
801 N. Fairfax Street, Suite 304
Alexandria, VA 22314
(800) 326-2642
www.counseling.org
Call or write for referral information about counselors in your area.

American Psychiatric Association
Public Affairs Office, Suite 501
1400 K Street, NW
Washington, DC 20005
(202) 682-6220
www.psych.org
For referral information about psychiatrists in your area.

American Psychological Association
750 First Street, NE
Washington, DC 20002
(202) 336-5800
www.helping.apa.org
Call or write for referral information about psychologists in your area.

Anxiety Disorders Association of America
11900 Park Lawn Drive, Suite 100
Rockville, MD 20852-2624
(301) 231-9350; (800) 545-7367
www.adaa.org
To obtain a list of mental health professionals who treat anxiety disorders or for a list of self-help groups in your area.

Association for Advancement of Behavior Therapy
305 Seventh Avenue, 16th floor
New York, NY 10001
(212) 647-1890
Call or write to request a list of mental health professionals in your state who use behavior therapy and/or cognitive-behavior therapy.

Emotions Anonymous International Services
P.O. Box 4245
St. Paul, MN 55104
(612) 647-9712

Freedom From Fear
308 Seaview Avenue
Staten Island, NY 10305
(718) 351-1717
www.freedomfromfear.org
Call or write for a free newsletter on anxiety disorders and a referral list of treatment specialists.

Healthy Place

www.HealthyPlace.com

The largest consumer mental health online site, providing comprehensive information on psychological disorders and psychiatric medications from both a consumer and an expert point of view.

National Alliance for the Mentally Ill

200 N. Glebe Road, Suite 1015

Arlington, VA 22201

(800) 950-NAMI

www.nami.org

Assistance in locating self-help groups in your area.

National Anxiety Foundation

3135 Custer Drive

Lexington, KY 40517-4001

(606) 272-7166

Provides referrals to NAF members and other mental health professionals around the country.

National Association of Social Workers

Clinical Registrar Office

750 First Street, NE, Suite 700

Washington, DC 20002-4241

www.naswdc.org

For referrals to qualified clinical social workers.

National Council on Alcohol and Drug Dependence

(800) 622-2255

www.ncadd.org

National Institute of Mental Health
(301) 443-4513
www.nimh.nih.gov
Latest on diagnosis and treatment of mental disease.

National Mental Health Association
1021 Prince Street
Alexandria, VA 22314-2971
(703) 684-7722; (800) 969-NMHA
www.nmha.org
Call or write for a list of affiliate mental health organizations in your area.

National Mental Health Consumers' Self-Help Clearinghouse
1211 Chestnut Street, Suite 1000
Philadelphia, PA 19107
(800) 553-4539; (215) 735-6082
www.libertynet.org/~mha/cl_house.html

National Self-Help Clearinghouse
25 West 43rd Street, Room 620
New York, NY 10036
(212) 642-2944

Psych Central
www.psychcentral.com
Online index for psychology, support, and mental health resources.

Recovery, Inc.
802 N. Dearborn Street
Chicago, IL 60610
(312) 337-5661

Self-Help Clearinghouse
Northwest Covenant Medical Center
25 Pocono Road
Denville, NJ 07834
(800) 367-6724 (in NJ); (201) 625-9565 (outside NJ)
www.cmhc.com/selfhelp/

## Nutrition

American Dietetic Association
www.eatright.org
Search here for a registered local dietitian.

Mayo Clinic Health Oasis
www.mayohealth.org
Articles on nutrition and virtual cookbooks.

Meals on Wheels Association of America
(703) 548-8024
www.mealsonwheelsassn.org
Locate Meals on Wheels in your area.

Tufts University Nutrition Navigator Nutritionists
www.navigator.tufts.edu
Reviews and rates Web nutrition sites.

## Obsessive-Compulsive Disorder

Obsessive-Compulsive Anonymous
P.O. Box 215
New Hyde Park, NY 11040
(516) 741-4901

Obsessive-Compulsive Foundation
P.O. Box 70
Milford, CT 06460
(203) 874-3843
www.ocfoundation.org

Obsessive Compulsive Information Center
2711 Allen Boulevard
Middleton, WI 53562
(608) 836-8070

## Panic

National Panic/Anxiety Disorder (NPAD) News
1718 Burgandy Place
Santa Rosa, CA 95403
(707) 527-5738
www.npadnews.com
Call or write for referral sources and contacts for support groups.

The Panic Center
Online support group and resources
www.paniccenter.net

Panic Support 4 U
An online support group for anxiety, panic, and agoraphobia.
www.Panicsupport4u.com

Season of Peace
Methods for finding relief from panic attacks, stress, and anxiety.
www.season.org

## PHOBIAS

Anxiety and Phobia Support Network
Help for those recovering from anxiety disorders.
www.anxietytofreedom.com

Anxiety and Phobia Treatment Center
The P.M. Newsletter
White Plains Hospital Center
Davis Avenue at East Post Road
White Plains, NY 10601
(914) 681-1038

Phobics Anonymous
P.O. Box 1180
Palm Springs, CA 92263
(619) 322-COPE
Over one hundred national groups.

## POSTTRAUMATIC STRESS DISORDER

Department of Veterans Affairs
Mental Health and Behavioral Sciences Service
810 Vermont Avenue, NW, Room 990
Washington, DC 20410
(202) 273-8431

International Society for Traumatic Stress Studies
60 Revere Drive
Northbrook, IL 60062
(847) 480-9028
www.istss.org

Patience Press
Information & Resources on PTSD
P.O. Box 2757
High Springs, FL 32655
(386) 454-1651
www.patiencepress.com

## Senior Resources

Access America for Seniors
www.seniors.gov
Government and agency services for seniors.

AgeNet
www.agenet.com
Information and referral network.

American Association for Geriatric Psychiatry
7910 Woodmont Avenue
Bethesda, MD 20814
www.aagponline.org
For referral to a geriatric psychiatrist, call (301) 654-7850 (ext. 100).

American Association of Retired Persons (AARP)
(800) 424-3410
www.aarp.org
Consumer group.

Eden Alternative
www.edenalternative.com
Living facilities with pets.

Eldercare Locator
(800) 677-1116
For local resources funded by Administration on Aging (AOA).


ElderCare Online
www.ec-online.net
An online community where peers and professional help improve quality
of life.


Elderweb
www.elderweb.com
Online eldercare sourcebook.


Medicare Hotline
(800) 638-6833
www.medicare.gov
Complete guide to Medicare.


National Academy of Elder Law Attorneys
(520) 881-4005
www.naela.com
Legal services to elderly and disabled.


National Council of Senior Citizens
(888) 373-6467
www.nclnet.org
Activist agency representing older Americans.


Older Women's League (OWL)
(800) 825-3695
Web site that focuses on women's issues.

SeniorLaw

www.senior.law.com

One-stop source for all legal matters affecting older people.

SeniorNet

www.senior.net.org

National nonprofit organization.

Visiting Nurses Association

(800) 426-2547

www.vnaa.org

## VOLUNTEERING OPPORTUNITIES

Administration on Aging

Department of Health and Human Services

200 Independence Avenue, SW

Washington, DC 20201

(202) 619-0724

www.aoa.gov

American Association of Retired Persons (AARP) Volunteer Center

(202) 434-3200

www.aarp.org

America's Promise

(800) 365-0153

www.americaspromise.org

Points of Light Foundation

(202) 729-8000

www.pointsoflight.org

Senior Corps

(800) 424-8867

www.seniorcorps.org

Federal agency for senior volunteers; offers a number of programs.

Senior Corps of Retired Executives (SCORE)

(800) 634-0245

www.score.org

VolunteerMatch

www.volunteermatch.org

Nonprofit online service that helps interested volunteers get involved with community service organizations throughout the United States.

# INDEX